Warm Hearts

A Nurses' Recipe for A Successful and Fulfilling Career

Not Just an Ordinary Nursing Book

Introduction

Ethics, Morals, and Kindness Went to the Dogs… I'm Cold as Ice

I reported to duty. It was my first day as a fully trained and certified nurse. I was prepared and confident in my sparkling white top and pants. (I could wear a skirt but no, I look better in pants and I wanted to look my best on my first day.) Do you want to know what else I reported with? I know you do not expect this considering what I said earlier, but, deep down, I was carrying fear and anxiety; a whole lot of it.

C'mon, don't say I wasn't ready. I swear I was. But imagine you were entering a hospital, not to be taken care of as you are used to, but to take care of and fix people without a friggin' idea of what they would come in looking like. And I'm not talking about their clothing or hairstyle. In nursing school, they told us to expect the worst. In my internship, I had seen the worst. However, I used my status as a trainee as an excuse to push the worst to the experienced (and certified) nurses. They would have to take it up because no one wanted themselves or the hospital on the spot, or the media poking their nosy noses if someone kicked the bucket because of 'mishandling'.

Now, it was different. I was already certified and armed with a little experience, so there were no excuses. I was going to see the worst and had to handle it myself. So, yes, I was so afraid and anxious because I did not know what kind of worst would walk through the door and if I could really handle it.

I had something else in my innermost being; a stone-cold heart. Don't jump into conclusions just yet; please let me explain. I know that they told you in school that you need to have a caring warm heart in order to get into a profession that requires you to take care of people in their worst. Nursing is one of those very noble professions.

I had that warm heart; I was considerate, empathetic, sympathetic, and compassionate, you name it. I mean, I had a deep love for people and I never would have been mean, ignorant or rude to anyone who needed my help. I was a simple person with a simple desire, the kind of person who made people's problems my problems and made it my business to make sure everyone was happy. I loved and felt loved, so I knew I would do very well in a field where I needed to care for people. That's why I chose to pursue nursing as a career.

So, where did the ice-cold heart I came to work with come from? It's a long, weird, and boring story but I'll give you the CliffsNotes version.

I was one of those students who did very well in the theory part of my education. However, I could not wait to get this bit over with and get to the practical part, which they told me is 'real' and exciting. Little did I know...

Either they forgot to tell me, were sparing my excited naivety or were just being selfish; they did not tell me about the scary, tearful, heartbreaking part. I had to handle real patients with real illnesses and injuries and emotions too. It was not the dummies I had gotten used to playing and 'talking' candidly with. Dummies never expressed pain or yelled, wailed, shed tears or gave me that pleading look that melted my heart.

The experience was not rosy. I cried a lot, mostly right in front of patients. I took on their emotions and suffering and actually made them my own. You can imagine absorbing all those people's emotions not to mention their suffering. It felt like I was suffering more than each individual patient.

Damn! Wasn't I an emotional mess? Eventually, I could no longer do my job properly. How could I attend to a person when I was in tears and suffering emotional breakdowns? I was supposed to be their shoulder to cry on, but... I was the emotionally unstable nurse who could not even stick a needle in a patient because they were winching in pain. To say the least, I was not of help to anyone. And I was not the only one; there were a few other 'noble souls' like mine.

The Magic Heart and Emotional Hack

Then we learned how to hack our emotions and 'soft' hearts, as they loved to call them. We deduced from our experiences and knowledge in this field that it was impossible to make it in this career with such soft and warm hearts. Hospitals were cold spaces and such a heart, your 'warm' energy would be sucked out.

Here are the few lessons we were taught:

- Patients needed medicine to get better and you need not get your emotions involved.
- You are not supposed to feel bad for anyone because you are not responsible for their suffering. So, empathy and even sympathy were out of the question.

- You needed not let people get to you; do what you need to and leave the rest to the universe. This translated to no mercy, no pity.

- No patient should tell you what to do because you are the professional and you know better how things should be handled. Which we understood as; we know everything and patients have no say. Whoever insists on dictating our work proves that they can treat themselves so let them be (ignore them).

- If you were friendly, people would take advantage and 'misuse' you. If you do not want patients, colleagues and basically everyone around your environment to take advantage, you need not have that friendly face. So, to succeed in my career, I was taught that friendliness would be a burden.

Being newbies, we believed that they knew better and we followed every technique in the book, about being cold, just like the hospitals should be so that nothing sucked at our energy – and we followed it like the gospel.

The Mega Transformation

So, this is how the warmth in my heart that I wanted to share with the world was turned cold as ice. I was told it was my weakness and that it would cause me pain and harm in my profession. They said nursing was a tough profession that would expose me to terrible situations and people in the worst of conditions. Such a tender heart that went out to all people just wouldn't cut it.

I remember I was once shouted at by my supervisor in a certain hospital where I was working as a trainee nurse hurling insults at me in front of patients! What had I done to earn that response? I was helping a patient fill out their medical insurance form. That supervisor said that if people were illiterate, it was not my problem; filling forms was not part of nursing and definitely not in my job description. True, it's not in my job description. But passed by and I saw them struggling and asking for help from others who turned a cold shoulder. I'd been heading to my room to idle around, because I did not have a patient to attend to at that time, so why not help? According to him, I should have hurriedly walked by as if I had an emergency case to attend to. But why pretend? (Of course I would not ask them that and risk termination so I just apologized and nodded.)

You would not guess my punishment for that 'mistake'. Since I was being so nice and idling around, they assigned me to the emergency room; I mean, who sends a trainee to an emergency room? I was told that there, I would find those who really needed my help and I could outdo myself helping around.

This is where I saw some of the scariest scenes I have ever witnessed in my career. Coincidentally I got in at a time when accident victims were just being received in the emergency wing. They were badly injured; it was so bad that some of them had limbs almost separated from their body. I hadn't been prepared to witness, let alone handle, such cases. People were wheeled in and the doctor in charge was yelling instructions. Patients wailed. One clutched at me. Yet another pleaded with me to save their child— laying just across them—first. Across from me, the doctor was yelling at me. (And here I thought we should keep calm in emergencies so as not to frighten the patients.)

I stood numb, rooted to one spot. I did not know what to do first or even last; everybody needed urgent help and I couldn't attend to everyone all at once. All that blood seemed to have dried mine up.

In the end, I chose to help the child first. Unfortunately, they died in my arms. My heart broke and tears flowed. I had failed. As if beating myself up was not enough, the doctor blamed me and said that I had mishandled the patients and that I had chosen not to listen to him because I wanted to be a hero. He even told everyone that the child was not badly injured and I should not have rushed to attend to them first. Of course, it didn't matter that some of the others had mere scratches; apparently, they could pay more. He did not forget to mention that I cried: I was "a useless, unprofessional crybaby."

Everyone I met—colleagues, janitors, and cleaners you name it— told me to toughen up and stop showing off. They said my kind of attitude would stress me to an early grave in these kinds of work environments. When I had worked in the hospital setting for a while, I started to believe they must know something I don't.

I Watched and Learned

It was this and a couple other similar incidents that froze my heart. Every morning, as I reported to duty, I reminded myself that I was there to give medical care and not to share my emotions or try to understand anyone else's. Patients needed medical care, not my heart.

I looked at how coldly other 'more experienced' colleagues behaved, and I emulated. I was there not only to learn nursing skills but also nursing attitudes. By the end of my residency, the nice kindhearted girl was gone and in her place was the smart nurse whose heart was cold as ice. She didn't give a crap about anyone. She was just there to do her job. Being nice was not in her job description. She was so stern-faced that no patient dared ask a question about how to care for their sick child, voice an opinion, or even have a conversation to better understand their condition. That's how she was told she would protect herself. And it seemed to be working.

So there, I reported to my new job armed with an ice-cold heart for my own sake. This was the attitude they told me would 'cut it'. I was there to do what I had to do, then go home to my family and collect my check every month.

Did it 'cut it'?

I have been a nurse for 20 years now. I am experienced, I have a good job, and I can say that what I wake up to do every day is fulfilling. It is worth the while. I love my job, I love my patients, and the hospital environment inspires me and gets me out of bed every day.

The question is, though: Did it 'cut it'? In other words, did the cold- hearted attitude get me this far? Does it make my job fulfilling? Does it get me through my tough days?

Cold Hearts and Bitchy Attitudes Do Not 'Cut It'

As you probably figured out by now, the cold heart and snobbishness did not cut it. It did not make my career or tough days any easier. Instead, it cut me into pieces. It is true that I no longer cried but, after 5 years, I was almost losing my mind. I had locked away every emotion that I wanted to let. I had watched people suffer when I could very easily have assisted them. I had been rude to patients who only wanted my help and did not deserve that response. I had even been mean to trainees.

I had slowly become a person caring not for people, or even myself, but for my job. I was a bad and selfish caregiver. The bad stares I got from those I was cold to haunted me every waking moment. The person I was deep inside did not agree with all this BS. I was not serving my divine calling; I was supposed to actually care for people.

So, yes, I almost lost my mind due to stress and frustration. I started hating my job and everyone involved with it; patients and colleagues alike. I was not happy and neither was anyone I rubbed shoulders with or attended to. I was in it for the money, for a career.

Unfortunately, most nurses are like me. I don't know what you might have heard about that sick attitude nurses walk around with, but I tell you that it's going to ruin peoples live, yours included.

I have made it through 20 years. It has not been easy; I still see and handle the worst and I still cry (not in front of patients, though). But instead of wallowing in pity, I have learned to pray for those who suffer. I have not it thus far because I hardened my heart. Trust me, if I still had that attitude, I wouldn't be here now. It's a warm heart and right attitude that helped me succeed in this career and made it worthwhile.

You chose this noble career so that you can help people. It may not be the main reason, but it was part of the reason, I'm sure. Now, if you want to be successful, to keep your sanity and fulfill your purpose, you must remain true to your calling. If you have met people who have derailed you like I did, then you sought help from the right place. I will tell and explain 5 values essential for every nurse and caregiver, values you must have in order to become a successful happy nurse and have the best outcomes in your career.

At the core of all these values, ladies and gentlemen, is a warm heart. In the nursing field, we learn the art of the warm heart to take care of ourselves and others so that everyone can be happy. Remember, as someone who has been on the opposite 'side', I am writing from experience. So, trust me when I say I know better. A warm heart is like a cup of hot chocolate on a cold rainy evening; warm, calming, and soothing to the soul.

That said, let us get started on creating warm hearts! I hope you enjoy it as much as you learn from it!

Table of Contents

1: A Good Attitude

I know you have great credentials; excelled in your studies and maybe graduated top of your class. These, and possibly a good aptitude, helped you land a good job, and that's great. There is something else, though, which will affect how your experience on the job and how long you could stay on: attitude.

We will get to that in a bit, but first, answer a few questions for me, will you?

Is everything going as you expected? I mean, you must have had some expectations about how your day-to-day activities and duties as a caregiver would go, right? Maybe you saw yourself attending to compliant from a humble patient desperate to get well. You would happily give care and then they would feel better, fall at your feet and thank you. It would be such a great feeling, wouldn't it?

I know my example is a little, you know, extreme but you envisioned something even if it's not as extreme. Have your expectations been met? Below is some truth about this thing called expectation.

The Challenge of Expectations Versus Reality

If you had an expectation similar at all to my example above, chances are, you didn't do your homework, buddy. In other words, you never did good research on the specifics of the environments your job would expose you to.

This's why you may find that your expectation is so grander and unrealistic. Of course, no matter how much homework you did, you can never get the real picture until you experience it.

You may have known that there will be small surprises, tiny deviations from your expectations that are easy to deal with. However, there are times when the reality turns out to be worlds away from your imagination and it becomes impossible to accept. In these cases, it's easy to lose it. You cannot stand their work environment and the requirements of your position. You badly want out, but...

There is No Other Choice

You have no other choice but to stay on. You can't have wasted all those years and loads of cash studying to come and quit. You have responsibilities back at home and you can't just walk out of a job. Where are you going to find another that pays just as much? As a result, the employer and the patients unknowingly have a caregiver who does not give a hoot about caregiving; you are just keeping a job.

It will not be as easy as you imagined

As you've learned—or will learn—the work of a nurse is not easy and the work environment is far from favorable. Working in the current health care system can be chaotic and very stressful, nothing like we envisioned. The reality may hit you so hard that you become someone totally different from the positive and caring person I know you are. It happened to me.

Surviving through Reality with Attitude

Don't wait for things to get easier, for the healthcare system to get better, or you may be waiting until the day you retire.

Yes, I said it. You may retire as a bitter nurse who never found joy in her job and who would be a good riddance for colleagues and patients alike. On the other hand, you could serve the best years of your life as a caregiver, enjoying and finding satisfaction in your work. You could be that nurse who patients ask for, colleagues yearn to work with. You will miss them and your absence will be mourned.

Those are your two options. Of course, everyone wants to be the latter, but the thing is, not many achieve it. It could be because they think it is impossible in such environments.

However, becoming the second option is not that hard. You only have to identify and harness the power of one very simple factor. It is one seemingly small thing that makes all the difference between these two outcomes. What's that factor? ATTITUDE!! You read that right. Attitude makes all the difference.

It is easy to think that so long as you show up and report to duty on time and carry out your responsibilities, your attitude doesn't matter. We can put on masks to hide our real feelings and moods, right? The truth, however, is that you should care about your attitude, perhaps more than you care about your looks, especially as a caregiver.

Yes, your attitude matters a whole lot!

Why Your Attitude Matters

Your attitude determines how well or badly you do everything, as well as the quality of your relationships. As a health worker, your attitude contributes a great deal to creating a professional healthcare setting for the sake of your patients and fostering a healthy work environment for your sake and that of other workers.

I know you face a lot of troubles and hardships in your line of work. It is easy for all the positivity to be drained from you. When I started out with positivity, they told me that my little 'all nice' me would be gone soon. True to their word, a few years on the job ushered me straight into the sulky rude nurse's party. The struggles and hardships had changed me, or so I thought.

Today, I know that no matter what I go through in my life and profession, nothing has the power to change me. A common saying goes, 'It does not matter what happens to you, what matters is how you respond to it.' Of course, we read it and thing, They say that because they do not have a freaking idea what kind of stuff I face every single day.

Trust me, whoever said those words knew exactly what they were talking about. They were referring to our little buddy (or foe, depending on how you use it) called attitude. Your attitude dictates how you perceive and react to circumstances.

What is attitude, though? Is it a feeling, an emotion? Let's find out.

Discovering Attitude

According to the dictionary, attitude is simply a way of thinking or feeling about something. It can also mean the same as one's perspective, point of view or approach.

Frank Freeman, however, defined it better. He says that attitude is "a dispositional readiness to respond to certain institutions, persons or objects in a consistent manner which has been learned and has become one's typical mode of response." (Emphasis mine.)

So, your attitude, whether good or bad, is an action or reaction that you have learned. It does not just happen; no circumstance can force an attitude on you. You have chosen to think in a certain way about something. In other words, your attitude is your doing; it's your choice to consistently think a certain way.

What Does Attitude Have to Do with Anything?

Winston Churchill said, "Attitude is a small thing that makes a big difference." This learned fellow was darn right!

The way you choose to think about or view things (again, I say this is your attitude) very much affects the choices you make regarding them. This is how you end up hating or avoiding someone or something without a definitive reason. It is safe to say that, if you really think about it, the real reason may sound like a very lame excuse.

For instance, if a health worker thinks a patient is a nuisance who's overacting to get attention or special treatment, can they really explain why they made that judgment? They are not in the patient's body to feel their pain, nor do they even know them well enough to be able to judge their character. The only explanation here is attitude; a very bad attitude, in fact. Their excuse is: They have seen it all before. The truth is, though, from previous experiences, they have conditioned their mind to think like that; they nurtured that attitude.

Components of Attitude

There are three components of attitude: the cognitive (mind), the emotional, and the behavioral.

The cognitive component: This is based on the information or knowledge about the person, job, or situation. You get this information from what you have heard about them, from experience, and so on. For instance, I received information that playing nice was not going to help me in my career.

The emotional component: This is based on how the information or knowledge that you have makes you feel. For instance, if you heard that giving injections is hard or you had a bad experience while giving them, you may become so afraid that you can never bring yourself to give an injection.

The behavioral component: This is based on how the information and feelings make you act or react. For instance, in our example above, your fear makes you never to try to inject anyone. Every time you are faced with a case where injections are involved, you make excuses to get your colleague to do it or you start yelling at a patient for not 'staying still' or wanting the injection yet it is you who has a problem.

That is how attitude, this very small thing, drives you to make choices or to behave. It starts with a seed (information) that is planted in a garden (the mind). The more you water it and give it nutrients (by referring to the information and feelings), the bigger it grows, and everyone can see the fruit (behavior).

So, ask yourself. What fruit are you bearing? Do you like it, and how is it affecting your life and those around you? If it's not serving you, you can always uproot the seed (challenge the knowledge/information or replace it) in the garden and carefully choose the one you want to plant, or change the nutrients you feed it. Once you have done this, you have yourself the fruit you desire.

Now, I hope you have finally understood what we are talking about here. Let's move on now that we are on the same page.

Types of Attitudes

We are breaking down everything there is about our little friend here. So, let's find out how many faces he wears.

Positive attitude

It pays attention to the good rather than bad in people, situations, etc. People wearing attitude are the kind of fellows who never see mistakes as setbacks. Instead, for every mistake, they see an opportunity to learn, to grow and a whole lot other positive stuff.

These people are likely to portray:

- Confidence
- Optimism
- Responsibility
- Resilience
- Willingness to adapt
- Humility
- Cheerfulness
- Flexibility
- Reliability
- Determinedness

Negative attitude

A negative attitude, on the other hand, turns a blind eye to the good and is a little sucker who is always looking for the bad in every person or situation.

Fellows with who wear this will likely complain about changes instead of adapting to them. Beware! They seek scapegoats to blame for their own mistakes/failures, too.

These people are likely to portray:

- Anger
- Pessimism
- Frustration
- Hatefulness
- Resentfulness
- Jealousy
- Inferiority complex
- Vengefulness

The neutral attitude

And now we come to the most confused of them all. The neutral attitude is a sucker that does not allow you to have a side. This is the one commonly referred to as the 'don't give a damn attitude'.

People who wear this attitude never give enough importance to anything or anyone. They look but never really see, listen but never hear. Even when they do see a problem, it's as if does not penetrate their consciousness. They will just ignore it and leave it for someone else who gives a damn to solve. And it never bothers them to do this.

Tell these people to change something and you will have to explain at length why they should. Yet, you would be wasting precious time; they do not see the need to change.

These people tend to manifest:

- Lack of emotion
- Indifference
- Detachedness
- Complacence

- Disconnectedness

Can Attitude Be Changed?

It is common to hear people say, "You cannot make me change. It's just who I am, it's my personality." Why did I mention this? Well, people confuse attitude and personality. Let's clear this up:

It's true that there is a very thin line between attitude and personality. They both make you behave the way you do but the former may change with different situations and experiences while the latter is more rigid and permanent. They say personality is as fundamentally you as your DNA; you can't change it, no matter how you try. On the other hand, attitude is learned and acquired. This means it can be unlearned.

Yes, it can

Yes, as mentioned, attitude can be unlearned or rather it can be changed. Remember, our attitudes come from experiences and also what we learn from the society. They are be based on are beliefs, whether they are true truth or merely perceives as true. Therefore, it is possible to change our attitude if we addressed their our beliefs.

How do you change your beliefs? You will need to address the three components of attitude we discussed earlier, which play a big role in creating beliefs.

The mental component: Change how you think. Check the thoughts that dominate your mind and intentionally choose the ones you want to entertain.

The emotional component: Change how you feel. I know that this can be a little hard. Emotions are messed up as hell as they are powerful and difficult to control. Sometimes they may feel like they want to take you over but with practice, effort, and mindfulness, you can be in control of them.

The behavioral component: Change what you do. You can do this easily if you learn to take a step back; to pause and have a second thought before you act.

Note: If the feelings start to get in the way, you can always rely on your thoughts and behavior to change an attitude. Do what you know is right, even if you do not feel like it in the moment. The feelings will have no choice but to follow suit.

There! That's the recipe for a good attitude. for you. Now, before you go and cook up anything, you must know this about attitudes: They have the power to build or destroy your life, your career, your outcomes and your mood every single day. So, be careful which one you carry around.

My advice? Choose the positive attitude. It has a good effect on everything; your behavior, character, life, career, family, and health. As Antoine de Saint-Exupery said, "The meaning of things lies not in the things themselves, but in our attitude towards them."

Now that we have a better understanding of what attitude is and how it affects us, we can discuss it in light of our noble nursing career.

Why Your Attitude As A Nurse Matters

There are a few reasons a nurse's attitude matters.

It affects your patient's attitude, thus their responsiveness and wellbeing

John Patrick, the author of Health Attitude: Unraveling and Solving the Complexities of Healthcare, states that 'the prescription starts with a single word, attitude.'

As a caregiver, your patients are affected by everything you do, and everything you do is determined by your attitude. When you walk around with a lousy mood because of some negative attitude you have, it will affect them negatively. Then, you will have already served them a negative/bad prescription.

Like a cold, attitude is contagious. This is especially true when it comes to patients. If you have a positive attitude, you will be surprised at how they glow and how much better they seem to be feeling because they feel that they have received care from a person who is concerned and has their best interests at heart.

On the other hand, with a bad attitude and rotten mood, you will see that everyone you come in contact with seems to get duller and wither. They will not like you offering any care to them because, even without saying anything, you communicate that you just do not give a damn. They can feel your coldness and have already 'caught' your attitude. No wonder you may be having harder days at work since you are likely to encounter more unresponsive, cold and rude patients. It's not that you are unlucky or people do not like you. Blame your attitude, my friend, because you will always get the taste of your own medicine.

It defines the quality of your services

We all know that you have very high qualifications but those were for school. On the job, they will not entirely determine your proficiency in giving care. Rather, your attitude weighs heavily here. You see, you may have all those good qualifications and recommendations but if your attitude does not match them, you will fail terribly in healthcare.

The think about it: If a bad attitude is clouding your day, you are more likely to make mistakes. It makes you careless and you will not be as attentive to your job. That's how you get cases of patients falling off theatre beds and medicines not administered in the right doses. I remember there was a time I was not attentive to a patient's weight before they were put on anesthesia and it took a great struggle to get them to wake up. They could have died.

You know very well that these kinds of mistakes are not acceptable in healthcare. You have been entrusted with people's lives. Where would you hide after a single deadly mistake?

Your attitude creates your working environment

How would you describe your work environment? Do you find it healthy or hostile? Your work environment is not about the buildings or decor; it's created by the people surrounding you, the state of the interpersonal relationships.

Your attitude towards people you work with, work for, and who you offer your services to determines the state of your relationship with them. It is obvious that a negative attitude will make your environment hostile, as you will find that you there is friction between you and colleagues, doctors and even patients.

If you cannot get along with people, that explains why your day gets screwed the moment you step into your workplace. I do understand that the hospital environment can be one of the worst. Sometimes, you can be too tired to play nice with everyone. But keep in mind that a hostile environment makes it even worse. So, why not try to keep an attitude that makes the environment a little bit easier to survive in? Trust me, it is good for everyone.

In Nursing, A Positive Attitude Is A Necessity – Not A Choice

Based on our discussion above, you should know that there is no room for negative attitude when it comes to healthcare. It really does not matter how bad the situation is, how you are feeling, or what wrong was done to you. You must have a positive attitude towards your employer, your work, your colleagues and other health workers, and your patients.

Do you remember the story I told you about being sent to the emergency room as just a trainee, unskilled and scared? What he did was not right, and it was just because he had a terrible attitude towards trainees. I mean, not only was I traumatized, but I could have mishandled patients. You have seen how it negatively affected me.

So, you decided to be a caregiver, right? So, check and manage your attitude. Often, if you find yourself being moody and mad most of the time in your practice, your attitude needs fixing. The following steps should help you fix any issues with your attitude issues so you can have one that befits your career and your calling to help others. I say it again: Nursing is not just a career; it's a calling.

How To Fix Your Attitude

1. Identify the Cause of Negative Attitude

We all leave nursing school positive, full of hope and big expectations of our careers. We are happy to report to work and more than happy to carry out our responsibilities. Positive attitude, check!

Then, something happens to most nurses, something unfortunate. Our attitudes change and we cannot stand the very patients that we swore to take good care of. We hate the workplaces we were once so anxious and excited to go to.

So, what happens? What changes our attitude for the worst?

- **Doubting your ability:**

Far too often, when you think your training got you prepared for everything and when you think you have everything figured out or you can handle anything, the realities you encounter prove you wrong. You try to solve issues but end up making a fool out of yourself. Sometimes, you aren't able to answer a patient's questions or reassure them. Some of them might be so rude as to ask if you really know what you are doing.

Because of such incidents when even you are not sure if you have a friggin' idea of what you are doing, you start to doubt your abilities and question whether you really made the right career choice. You lose belief in your ability to handle cases, even the simplest ones. You convince yourself that you are a dunderhead in a nurse's uniform you do not deserve to wear, all because of a few blunders. You start to avoid your duties, making excuses why you cannot attend to them. Gradually, resentment for everyone and everything that is related to your job sets in. Your attitude towards your work has changed because you believe you are incapable of doing it right.

- **Friction with a coworker**

It is inevitable that in any workplace, there will always be a villain. This person seems to be hell-bent on ruining your day and making your work difficult.

Have you encountered this person (or people)?

In my case, it was that doctor who sent me to the emergency room, blamed me for a death and later badmouthed me to the whole hospital! After that incident, I hated every waking day of my internship. He completely turned my attitude on its head. A person like that could greatly contribute to a negative attitude.

- **Burnout**

Maybe you have been on the job for a long time and have fallen into a boring routine. It seems like you wake up to do the same thing every day and it's become exhausting. Most are the times you wish that something would change. As a result, you are no longer the same caring and attentive nurse who started out. Now, you are a grumpy, tired nurse who is desperately hoping for change and who sees their job as a liability and patients a nuisance. You feel like you are 'trapped' at this job and your good attitude has been adversely affected.

It's normal to feel this way after years of working at the same job every single day. These feelings are as a result of burnout. This is categorized as physical, mental, and emotional exhaustion and disengagement. Many confuse it with stress but it is important to note that being stressed and experiencing a burnout are two very different states. Stress is associated with over-engagement; when you have to run up and down involving your mind, emotions and body in everything such that at the end of the day you are overwhelmed. On the other hand, burnout is associated with disengagement; you just aren't as involved. Your body is present, but your mind and emotions are long gone. Even your physical is 'refusing' to be there – like really be there.

Causes of burnout

This disengagement is not caused by job demands or the fact that you have to come do the same job every day. I mean, most of us don't change job every other year and most any job does makes too many demands, and yet not everyone experiences burnout. No, burnout is the result of too many job demands, inadequate resources, and little recovery.

Let me expound on that:

- ✓ Job demands are the aspects of your work that require you to put in continuous effort and energy. That's why they drain you. They involve things like emotionally demanding interactions with colleagues and patients, big workloads and the high pressure they come with, role conflict etc.

- ✓ Job resources consist of the components of the work environment that reduce the sting of job demands, foster growth and learning, and help you achieve your job goals. They include high quality relationships and interactions, opportunities to learn new things and grow, support from the leadership, positive feedback, autonomy, etc.

- ✓ Recovery refers to the breaks that you take after work or when you are off duty; whether it's at night or during the day after your shift ends, during weekends and during vacations. You can recover by doing things that uplift your soul or stuff that you enjoy which should help you release some steam. They help you get back to work reset and refreshed.

Signs of burnout

- ✓ A negative attitude towards work
- ✓ Dulled emotions; that moodiness/awful feeling is a very good example
- ✓ Lack of motivation and a sense of hopelessness; you start to feel ineffective on the job
- ✓ Chronic exhaustion; you are worn out and extremely fatigued, even if you just reported on duty an hour ago
- ✓ Irritability; you are like a ticking time bomb with buttons out waiting for a little push from anyone to explode

- **Stress**

As I mentioned earlier, the work of a nurse is not easy, not at all. You have to deal with people at their worst and somehow find a way to make them feel better. Chances are, you may develop compassion fatigue, a type of stress that comes from caring too much for others. It comes as a result of absorbing other people's suffering out of empathy. It's only natural when you listen to their sad stories and watch their pain filled faces. This kind of stress is a heavy load on your mind and body. In the long run, your work environment may become a place you loath because it stresses you out. When that's the case, a negative attitude has already set in and you cannot stand the place or the people.

2. Handle the Triggers

The triggers of negative attitude discussed above are normal; they can happen to anyone. The problem is not the triggers, it is how we respond to them. So here is how we can address the discussed triggers;

- **Create better relationships**

✓ Try to get along with everyone

Good healthcare is the product of team effort, which is only possible in a healthy working environment. It is important that a nurse keeps a good and collaborative relationship with colleagues and other healthcare staff. I am not implying that it is possible to get along with every single person; there's always a colleague who is a pain in all the wrong places. However, even if you don't like or can't stand them, put your work as a caregiver before your feelings and check your attitude so you can work together.

Also, relating well with your patients (even though they can be difficult) will help create a healthy working environment. You see, when you maintain a positive attitude towards a difficult patient, they will feel your care and genuine concern and eventually, they will ease up and be more likely to speak up or cooperate. This way, they make your work easier, which leads to positive results. Also, you will not be as unhappy at the end of the day; the mere fact that you impacted someone's life positively will make all the trouble worth the while. There is no better way to vamp your mood!

- **Prevent burnout**

    ✓ Put yourself first

You were told that as a caregiver, you ought to put everyone's needs before yours. Nurses are notorious for their selflessness. In their quest to care for others, as their job (and calling) demands, they think of themselves last or not at all. This puts them at risk of burnout.

Putting yourself first can be very useful in combating this risk. In my 20+ years of experience on the job as a nurse, I have learned that as I tend to other people, I should first learn to tend to myself. You need to love yourself so you can have love and care to give. If you do not put you first, you become a slave to your patients, your work, your colleagues, you name it. Everyone and everything will drain you, leaving you empty and sad.

✓ So, you have to know when enough is enough, when to step aside and let God, when to readjust and care for self. Put yourself first.

✓ Engage in an activity you love at least once every day to keep your joy

- ✓ Make your mental, physical, spiritual, and emotional health a priority by scheduling intentional time to relax the body, soul and mind.

- ✓ Get enough sleep.

- ✓ Since you are called to give, rather than being selfless giver (who gives all without regard for their own needs), be an otherish giver (one who gives but finds a way to balance their giving with self-care and self-interest). This means you can give, but you never give so much that you leave yourself dry and burned out; you give also to yourself.

- ✓ Prioritize nutrition. Nursing is a demanding profession. The tasks you have to do every single day are energy suckers. This is why you have to ensure that whatever you eat provides healthy fuel for the body to run on. It will help you keep going and it's usually easier to manage stress on a full stomach and a healthy mind and body. You do not want your body to be trying to manage a sugar rush while trying to balance cortisol levels.

- ✓ Find and engage in a hobby unrelated to your career

Although you chose to be a healthcare worker, I am pretty sure there are other things you can do very well. Granted, you may not realize it since you spend all your darn days working and your nights asleep on the couch in your day's clothes, you have some other natural talents.

Pay more attention to yourself and what you love to do (when you are not judging yourself so harshly) and you will see them. They are your passions and you ought to create time to tend to them.

How does this help with burnout? Well, engaging in that hobby activates a different part of your brain and gives a rest to that which takes care of the nursing work. It helps you challenge your brain in different ways and provides you with new knowledge and (don't forget) it's fun, too. This way, nursing does not become the only life and knowledge you have.

- **Manage stress**

Your work will be stressful; you cannot avoid that fact. However, you can develop ways to cope, manage and release the stress. The following tips will help you:

✓ Adopt a 'brain dumping' practice

You take on a lot every day. From patients crying out in pain and relatives fussing, to people dying right in front of you despite all your frantic efforts to save them. The mental strain is enormous and real. If you let it stay, it will seep into other areas of your life. As a result, you will not have a life outside your work environment. Eventually, it can become quite overwhelming and it is likely to negatively affect your career and your mental wellbeing.

To avoid this, adopt a brain dumping process. Here is how it works:

Upon getting home, set a timer for around 20 minutes and take this time to go over your day in your mind and write about it on a piece of paper. Don't be formal, as if you are writing a report; you are allowed to use any language and any word that could best describe the events for you. (Yes, you can write about the annoying dumb as a goat supervisor.)

When the timer goes off, pick up the piece of paper and without reading it, crumble it and toss to the dustbin. Why should you never read it? Because laying it all on paper was meant to upload it from your brain thus reading it would be reloading it all back. And you know the brain will start fussing and analyzing everything, adding to your stress. When that's done, you can now go soak in the tub, take a shower, or whatever else you do to unwind and relax. But I advise you take a bath fist to freshen up.

The brain dumping process helps you keep work stress (which is unavoidable) from spilling into your life outside of work. Also, it freshens up your mind so you're ready for tomorrow's stress. All this leaves you less likely to overload.

- ✓ Take time for yourself

We may not all have the means to go to tropical islands but we all have ten minutes to spare. Tony Robbins, an excellent life coach, is of the opinion that "if you do not have at least ten minutes for yourself, you do not have a life."

So, always set aside 'me time' to unwind and do something that helps you feel relaxed; something that helps keep you grounded. It could be yoga, meditation, retail therapy, listening to music, having a nature walk, what have you.

Bottom line is: Take good care of yourself. If you do not take care of you—your mental, physical, and emotional you—then you will not be able to take care of anyone else. You will age in this noble career in the most terrible way, and you will be blaming everyone for it when you're the one to blame. Take care of you first, then you will have the mental capacity, the emotional balance, the strength, and the perfect attitude to take good care of others, and love doing it.

3. Create A Positive Attitude

After hacking negative attitude triggers, you will need to adopt an attitude that will finally kick the negative to the curb, once and for all. Otherwise, it may just hide somewhere in your being and crop up every now and then. (You know what they say about kicking out one demon; you need to fill the void; otherwise, it will wander around and come back with seven others only to come back to find its house clean, empty and welcoming.)

As we discussed earlier, a positive attitude is the best kind. Mind you, just because it's good, doesn't mean that it's automatic. No, my dear; a positive attitude will not come as easily as they tell you it will. You must create or rather cultivate it, and this is not going to be an easy process. Don't worry so much about it, though. We're going to break down the process. I believe you can nail it.

i. Realize that you are in charge and can control your attitude, and how you respond to circumstances, environments or people, which you can't control.

The first step is to realize and get it in your beautiful mind and embrace the fact that you have all the power when it comes to your perception of things: your attitude. It is not influenced by what happens to you or who does what, but emerges from how you decide to interpret it. Consider the following example:

Three girls receive a fancy gift from a guy friend. The first one thinks, He's so thoughtful. The second one, He's such a showoff, he wanted to show me he can afford this stuff. The third one, He's trying to buy me out with a watch!

You see? They all interpreted a simple gift differently; and their reactions will be follow suit. No. 1 may hug him, No. 2 may sneer, and No. 3 may throw it at his face. Their attitudes control their reactions.

This clearly tells us that your attitude is your choice. You are holding the steering wheel of the car headed towards your attitude. You choose where to park; negative, positive, or the confused neutral location.

ii. Check your mind

What's in your mind? There are thoughts, which in turn create beliefs, which in turn affect the way you interpret things? Positive and strong beliefs create favorable environment for a positive attitude to grow while negative and weak beliefs do the opposite.

I will use a family at the dining table as our example:

Situation: The daughter comes in with 3 friends just when dinner has been served. She had not announced she would be having guests for enough food to be prepared; she just showed up.

As a mother, you might think:

Negative/weak belief: This girl never does anything right. Does she think this is a restaurant, or what? And those friends lack manners. How do they come here like this? They are a bad influence on my daughter.

As a result, you then serve dinner with a long face and keep giving your daughter and her friends dirty looks from across the table. Tension can be felt in the room and food is hardly going down people's throats.

Strong and positive belief: They came unannounced but who knows what the situation could have been for them to come here like this. We'll just share the food; everyone will have a bite. As a result, everyone enjoys dinner as there is a lot of chitchat knowing her friends and enjoying the food.

You see, the same event can be framed in two different ways. You must create beliefs that portray events in a positive way, even when it's a negative event. As they say, "Try to see the good in everything." It sounds crazy but, in every situation, there is always something positive. Your ability to see the silver lining is determined by what you choose to see or rather how you choose to look at or thing about it.

So, if you want to cultivate a positive attitude, start by cultivating positive thoughts, which will then become your beliefs. You will see how it is possible to see an insult by a patient in a positive light. They may call you incompetent, but instead of lashing back you smile because you think, At least they can speak, or, That's better than holding it in and cursing me inwardly, or, Not such a bad accusation. At least I can defend myself by giving good care to prove my competence. All this is because you do not carry around a belief that patients are a nuisance, but that they are people with feelings and who sometimes can talk nonsense they do not mean.

iii. Enrich yourself with positivity

You must realize that how strong negativity is. It's like the stench of garlic; you have to use other spices just to cover it up. This is how negative thoughts, beliefs, events, etc. are compared to the positive. For this reason, you have to saturate yourself with positivity in all areas of your life and in every manner possible to counter them when they come. Below are a few examples how:

Enrich your mind with positive thoughts by reading, viewing, or listening to some inspirational or motivational content before you go to bed and as part of your morning routine. This ensures that you go to sleep and open shop engulfed in positivity. My personal favorite was a motivational talk by Les Brown.

Stay away from negative media. People in mainstream media and social media seek publicity by selling propaganda meant to make innocent people paranoid, unhappy, and afraid. It's incredible how this kind of crap hooks people. If you keep exposing yourself to stuff in the media that affects you negatively, all the positivity you have been trying to build will be eroded.

My recommendation: Avoid any media content that goes against what you believe in. You may 'just be watching', as we like to call 'indiscriminative watching', but your subconscious mind (the one that keeps a record of everything you experience to create your beliefs) is taking note. Do not give it a second glance if you come across anything like that; give all negative media a complete blackout.

iv. Keep close to those with positive vibes and keep your distance from naysayers

There are people who see the world through crap-colored glasses; the naysayers. Even in good situations, they have an eye for the negative in it, and they never shy away from saying it out loud to take someone off cloud nine.

No one seems to have figured out what wrong with those party poopers, so even with your good heart and intentions, do not try to 'make them see the light'. Instead of pulling them into your light, they are more likely to pull you into the dark – somehow negativity and darkness are way too powerful.

The other day, one of those friends I've never met but are somehow 'fam' on social media (I bet you have some) sent me a common quote I found very odd, but which made a lot of sense. It goes, "Never argue with a stupid (read: negative) person. They will bring you down to their level and beat you with experience." So, leave them alone. Maybe you work in the same department and you cannot avoid them entirely. However, you should make your contact very minimal.

Who do you stay around, then?

Make sure that your inner circle is made of people with whom you share common beliefs and who are looking for the good in everything. Vibes are contagious. If you are friends with a person with positive vibes, somehow you tend to catch them.

I have this friend who keeps me in the positive even when it feels like my life has been turned upside down. They use an all-time classic, "Everything happens for a reason, a good reason." With this mantra, I have seen myself approach sticky situations with a positive outlook and saved my eyes some tears and my mind unnecessary stress. These are the kind of people you need around you for that positive attitude to grow and flourish.

v. Mind your mouth—Positive output only!

It's likely that you have heard the statement 'words have power'. It does not sound serious or rather heavy, does it? Maybe that's why most of us do not take words seriously. What's the result? We screw up our own realities by the words we carelessly throw around.

They say that your mouth's output reflects what's in your brain. That's true. Do you know what else is true? Your words program your brain how to think. Talk positive, and your brain learns that it should think the same way.

For instance, when I first got assigned to the theatre, I had quite a crappy attitude about the place thanks to the negative stories I had heard. I seemed to mess up everything and was almost convinced I could not handle it, until one good doctor offered a 'cure' through a brief conversation.

It seemed as if he saw my frustration one day while I was handling a task. His approach made me stumble and stammer because I thought he had come up to me because I was certainly doing something wrong. I expected some berating but he just asked me to step back and breathe. I obeyed. Then, he asked, "Do you want to do this? Do you believe you can?"

"Absolutely," I replied.

The simple statement that followed has made a great impact in my life today. He told me, "Tell yourself what you just told me."

I have to say that it did not make much sense then, but I tried it anyway. I said to myself, "I believe that you can do this. It's hard but you are capable. You got this." It's hard to explain how these words affected me but I can tell you that I used them every time negativity overtook me and I felt like I could not do something, and somehow I would keep going until I finished the task. My mind was no longer that little bitch sabotaging me; it cooperated. This is how I confirmed that what you say to yourself has a lot to do with how you think.

We mind our vocabulary when talking to others but it's time we paid that kind of attention to the vocabulary we use when talking to ourselves. If you want to have a positive attitude, use positive vocabulary.

So, when you hit a snag, experience difficulty and get angry, do not use negative phrases such as "I can't," "I suck at this,'" "This won't work," "I am so damn mad,' "I am so clumsy," etc. Say, "I can," "I can try one more time," "It is doable," "I am a little upset, I need a break," etc.

When they ask, "How are you?" or "How your day is going?" do not say, 'I am hanging in there," or, "Just okay." Say, "It's terrific, never been better," or the Les Brown classic "Better than best, better than most." These words were used by a patient who lost all mobility due to an illness. She said it to those who visited her in the hospice, when they expected her to be 'hanging in there'.

Final thoughts on attitude: Your attitude is as a result of your choices, your thoughts, your beliefs, and your words. If you want to make it positive, you need to address all those areas. A positive attitude will make your life and even work experience better than best. Even in the hardest of times, you will pull through. People and even you will be surprised at how you thrive, how better you treat people and approach your job and even how your productivity increases. Every other principle would not matter or even work without attitude. It is the main ingredient; without it, everything else would be tasteless and meaningless.

2: Compassion
What Is It to Have Compassion?

When can we say that a person has compassion or is compassionate? Well, it is when they possess an ability to understand the emotional state of another person as well as their own.

There is more, though, a catch. Call it its unique flavor: A big part of being compassionate involves being less 'judgy' and having a different perspective when it comes to your perception of others – and the things they do or say.

What is the common perspective? People like to jump to conclusions and only perceive things based on surface appearances, which often is. The different perspective of a compassionate person looks deep beyond the surface, gives the benefit of a doubt and is patient.

Let me explain using a real-life example: Say you meet your neighbor with his son on your way to the grocer. You haven't seen them for a while and wish to catch up. You say hello, they say hello back, but they don't stop to say anything else. They don't even seem to be paying any attention to you. You mumble, "It's been a while," trying to get a conversation started but they walk away as if they never heard a word you said. So, you stand there, mouth agape, wondering what you ever did to them to be snubbed in such a way. You thought you were besties!

What would any person immediately think or say about the situation?

The ordinary person would think that the neighbor has developed a snobbish attitude, one they will most definitely associate with some material possession they acquired recently. They would talk of how insulted they felt and bad mouth them to others.

What Would a Compassionate Person Do?

A compassionate person, on the other hand, would not be so quick to judge and talk ill of the neighbors. They would not jump to conclusions and assume the worst. Instead, they would think that there must be a good reason for the behavior. A compassionate person understands that a person can do something, which seems okay to them, but which irritates others or seems inconsiderate and rubs others the wrong way unintentionally. They know that the neighbor did not mean to snub them and even if it were so, there must be a good reason, which they can enquire about later.

The Truth of The Situation as They Later Find Out is

It turns out the neighbor's son lost all the money meant to buy groceries for a week on his way to the grocery store. They were pre- occupied searching for it, afraid and angry that all that money could be lost. Their eyes and emotions were engaged, and they could not pay attention to you. They did not mean to offend you. If you ask them, it could be that they did not notice whoever said hello; they do not know it was you!

So, if you evaluate our scenario above, who handled the situation better? Is it the ordinary man or the compassionate man? You be the judge, but my take is the compassionate man did best.

Unfortunately, most of the time, we act as the ordinary man. We tend to assume the worst and end up treating people very badly. I know that not everyone means well but it is best to assume the best, understand peoples' suffering and try to do something about it. It makes the world a better place if we are compassionate.

And when it comes to healthcare, particularly as a nurse, compassion plays a very major role in determining the quality of healthcare given and also the satisfaction of all parties involved. Given the kind of environment they work in, it is safe to say that compassion is one of the basic ingredients to making things work well for everyone.

Compassion in Nursing

The kind of compassion required in the world of nursing does not only involve being aware of the other person's feelings. Called compassionate care, it involves understanding/relating to how they feel and doing your best to enable them to retain their wellness, independence and dignity.

Compassion for Patients

It cannot be emphasized enough that compassion is a key ingredient in the nursing profession. Without it, you may as well quit and go home because you are not of any help to anyone; neither yourself, your colleagues, nor your patients.

Let me tell you a story of a patient (who happens to be my niece) who knows too well what compassion can do:

It had been a year since she lost her pregnancy and the bleeding had not stopped yet. She went to the doctor and was advised to get some tests to check what the heck was going on with the yearlong bloody catastrophe. Several tests later, the doctor could not find anything wrong other than imbalanced hormones. He gave her a prescription for it and she went home hoping to get better. Two months later and after the medicine was finished, there still was no positive change. She went back to the doctor and would have to go back many other times because none of the prescriptions given seemed to work.

Due to the many visits, nurses and other staff around the hospital had gotten accustomed to her. She once heard one who was tasked with ensuring her tests were done terming her as 'the bleeding lady' when asked by a colleague the name of the patient. What a disgusting name! How callous can some people be!

This hurt so much but not more than the day she was waiting for her results and a cluster of nurses chitchatting seemed to take forever to avail themself to her. Rather annoyed for being kept waiting by gossiping nurses, she demanded their attention, stating that she was running out of time and needed to get this over with and go back to work.

The nurse in charge looked at the result sheet and said to her with a sneer, "Madam, leave that work alone. You do not have many days remaining for it anyway." Before my niece could recover from that venom, and figure out what exactly she meant, more was poured. “It says you have cervical cancer, at stage two. Few survive that.” She then shoved the paper to my niece and did not give her further explanations, directions or even attention. The nurse had just given her the most heartbreaking and life changing news and yet she did not seem to give a hoot about the patient, her condition and how to break such heartbreaking news about her condition.

The nurse just went on chatting without giving her a second look.

To this day, my niece tears up when she talks about how the news of the disease, which robbed her of the ability to become a mother at a tender age, was broken to her. It was in such a callous manner that she felt like someone had hit her hard in the chest, collapsing her lungs. She sat there panting, her head pounding. All this while, the nurse in question did not pay attention to her to notice her distress.

Fast forward, many months later throughout her treatment: She has met many nurses. Most of them are good to her, though some are indifferent, just doing their job. However, she recalls one particular nurse with red hair who attended to her during the time she was undergoing radiotherapy and was losing her hair, her vibrant skin, and sense of taste.

Everything tasted like steel. She says she was not very worried about her uterus; she was far more worried about her skin and the hair she was losing! She was a social figure on TV and the possibility of losing her looks would be quite a big blow to her livelihood.

You can see her face light up when she tells of how the red head once brought a head scarf and made a stylish head wrap out of it, applied make up and made her take pictures even though she did not want to because in her mind, she knew how awful she looked. She was amazed when she peeked at the pictures and even posted them online for her fans to catch up with her recovery. She was so beautiful. She still looked amazing. Being a woman who made such a fuss about her appearance, this really affected her positively. It gave her confidence and the will to fight the disease because, as she says, she felt that she "still got it!"

The nurse friend was just doing this out of kindness and to lift her mood by making her laugh a little. However, she did not know that, with her seemingly small action, she had helped restore the confidence of a young woman who thought that her life was over, who did not have the strength to face the world after all those treatments. She had just given hope to a patient who was giving up on herself. It was that day that she stopped letting the illness take her and started to fight alongside the medication with a strong will and positive expectation, simply because someone had reminded her that she still got it!

While she will never forget or even stop tearing up when she talks of the inconsiderate nurse who gave sensitive information so callously and predicted a impending death, she will also never forget the love, care and compassion she got from a young red- haired nurse who had a great impact in her journey fighting cancer.

My niece's healing is miraculous. According to her, she would be long dead if one person, a caregiver whose job description never involved tying head wraps or applying makeup and taking pictures, had not gone out of their way and did something for her out of compassion; something that changed the lenses through which she viewed her life. It was a change that gave her the strength to fight.

So, as you can see from my niece's story above, compassion counts a great deal. It has the power to heal, to give hope and to encourage. It will make a huge difference in the lives of those you serve.

Kindness, the Hallmark of Compassion

We've been talking about compassion so far, but perhaps it would be more clearly understood if we use a related, almost synonymous, word: kindness.

What does it mean to be kind towards others?

To be kind to a person is basically about paying attention to them, acknowledging their point of view (even if it does not mirror yours) and trying to understand their situation. It is a sort of understanding that conveys openness without judgment, ensuring that the other person's dignity is respected.

Unkindness, on the other hand, is failing to demonstrate understanding, judging people and their situations and blocking openness. There is nothing good about being unkind, obviously, but why do we find it to be the common trait among health care workers?

Why most people want to be unkind

It is a sad truth that even though nurses can be kind and are aware of what good that can do, they choose to be unkind to colleagues and patients alike. This is why:

- ✓ To protect themselves; it prevents people from getting 'too close'

Instead of bringing peace, joy and togetherness (which brings people close), unkindness encourages difference and separateness. It creates a wedge between 'us' and 'them'. Have you walked into situations where you can already feel the separateness? Like you and the others are standing on two opposite ridges with a deep, cold river in between?

Did you feel welcome, even to voice a greeting or display a smile let alone explain your situation or give an opinion? I'm certain you did not.

This is how the 'caregivers' want their patients to feel. They do not want them to overstep boundaries and get too close. It is true that it can become mentally and emotionally draining to listen to people's problems and suffering all day and connect with them in a way that you want to make them feel better.

It is not one of the best feelings; a nurse who has gone through this struggle may want to keep people from getting that close and may result in unkindness. Are you doing this, slowly turning your heart to into a block of ice?

- ✓ They want to feel superior and in control

A nurse who wants to be the one calling all the shots, especially if they are in a senior position, will use unkind tendencies to maintain power/control over the other person, whether it is over a patient or colleague. This nurse wants to ensure that the other person knows their place. They are very afraid that their kindness will be perceived as weakness and people will not obey or respect their authority.

I recall that they told me I was playing too nice and that I would be taken advantage of, so I had to become unkind. Deep inside, though, I was just afraid that I would not be respected or that I would be found wanting.

What does unkindness birth?

- ✓ Effective communication is hindered

Most of the times, patients do not receive the care they need because they can already sense that they are in the 'them' lane. There is no openness; they feel no freedom to communicate their thoughts or concerns about their health.

The same is true for colleagues. There is separation and bullying in what is supposed to be a supportive profession. Given how tough we all have it, we are all need mutual support.

- ✓ The quality of healthcare is affected

When communication is affected, the quality of healthcare is affected as well. This is why modern healthcare has transitioned from the traditional 'caring for patients' to simply 'prescribing a cure, no strings attached' kind of healthcare. As a result, there are endless stories being told about the many failures of the healthcare system.

We have become a society that values self-promotion more than connection with others. We have ignored humane qualities needed in healthcare and preferred to make perceive people as measurable targets.

Kindness Wins Any Day, Every Day

Kindness will calm and warm your heart and those of others who come into contact with you.

The importance of kindness in healthcare

- ✓ It keeps unnecessary and unwanted stress at bay

The people associated with healthcare facilities (patients, nurses and other healthcare workers), are a sensitive, scared and stressed lot. While patients are suffering due to illness, the nurses and other healthcare personnel are suffering due to the stress from their demanding jobs. Kindness would surely do everyone some good. Plus, if we stop being mean to each other, we get rid of yet another source of stress.

- ✓ Communication gets better

Kindness makes communication easier for all parties. For instance, there are patients who have to go through embarrassing and undignified procedures, or talk about messed up personal feelings. These types of people are quite vulnerable. They will not open up as supposed if they feel a barrier between you. Kindness makes them feel safe. It relaxes both them and the caregiver.

There may be some tension as none of them knows where to begin the conversation. However, where kindness is present, the tension is felt and acknowledged and defused. After all, it is easier to say, "I'm scared," or, "I really don't know where to begin," to someone who does not have unkindness plastered on their sneering face. Then, there is a greater chance that beneficial conversations will take place.

The Basics of Kindness

i. Listening to someone and understanding their situation. Once you've done this, you can challenge or support them to move on from it. However, it is important to understand that not all situations will require that kind of action.

ii. Leaving things as they are, not imposing your ideas, opinions or agendas. Watch and look for nonverbal (and even verbal) signals to know whether they are in need of or your opinions or even advice. For instance, when a patient under your care passes on and the family is mourning, wailing etc., sometimes they will blame you for not doing enough. The best thing you can do is let them be; no opinions, no defense, and no interference.

iii. Treating others as you would love to be treated is one of the best ways you learn how to show kindness to others. I have not known a soul that is unkind to themself.

So, before you act towards a person, focus on them and imagine what it would be like to be them at that point and time. How would you like to be treated? Consider your answer and act in the same manner.

How to Be A Compassionate Nurse

- ✓ Offer a listening ear to your patients

Listen to them when they talk about their issues or when they are presenting complaints. It can greatly improve their situation if a patient feels that you are actually listening rather than hearing them to give a prescription. It also helps put you in a better position to understand them and give appropriate care.

You see, sometimes patients will not know how to express themselves well. However, when you listen keenly, you will be able to pick up on symptoms and feelings that they may not be aware of or which they do not know how to express.

✓ Have positive vibes only

Strive to be positive throughout your interactions with patients, their relatives, and your colleagues. Projecting this warmth makes people feel close to you; they tend to be more comfortable around you. You should not only show it through your words or action but also with your body language, too. The following non-verbal cues (body language) will help you achieve the compassionate look:

- Smile. Be mindful of the occasion, though. (You don't smile when standing over a dead body, giving relatives the sad news, do you?)

- Apply a kind tone to your voice. It soothes.

- Make eye contact. It portrays honesty, respect, trustworthiness, and a sense that the conversation is important to you. People want that when they place their lives in your hands.

- Maintain your calm in emergencies, even when you know things are messed up real bad.

- Nod occasionally when you understand. It shows that you are actually following and encourages them to keep going.

  ✓ Socialize

They may have told you that you are here to work, not to make friends or make conversation. However, good and compassionate healthcare requires that you make friends and have those open conversations with your patients.

In one word, socialize!

Get to know your patients beyond their illness. You can begin with knowing their interests. Since you are not homies or besties, you will not go up to them and say, "Hey, what are your interests?" If you do not want to come off as the queer nurse rather than the friendly one, use the following approach:

Start the conversations by sharing about your own interests and see if they reciprocate by giving a signal that they want to talk about such stuff. They may tell you about theirs or just listen intently, wanting to hear more about you. This signals that they are ready to roll. You can then go ahead and ask them about their interests, hobbies or families, if they haven't told you yet. Get them talking about anything that is comfortable to talk to. Ask them about their day and if you have time, spent some of it with them, chit-chatting.

Socializing with patients makes them to feel more comfortable around you. Even as you assist them with the embarrassing stuff— such as having to bathe a grown man— the conversation will help them not to feel like a burden. It also helps you know them a little bit more so you can figure out how to better take care of them and make them feel more at home and at ease. For instance, if you know a patient loves to read, you can bring books for them or read to them if they are unable to do it for themselves. You could also turn on their favorite TV shows as you feed them. Trust me, this level of detailed care works wonders. And it's all thanks to socializing.

- ✓ Check in on them regularly

Patients often shy from asking for your help, even when they need it, especially patients who cannot perform the basic duties for themselves. In my experience, they start feeling like they are too needy and a burden to others. It becomes even worse if you see them that way, too.

This is where your 'silent' compassion is needed. You can go out of your way to check in on them quite regularly and see if they need any help. They may have a request or a concern that they may have not had anybody attend to, or maybe they were afraid they would bother you since you seemed so busy. So, as you do your tasks, stop by your patients' rooms and ask them if they need anything in particular. You could get someone a glass of water to take their medication or adjust a pillow.

It may seem like a lot of work on top of your already hectic schedule, but this kind of thoughtfulness is worth your while. It will help build strong bonds with your patients. Also, people seem to feel better and be happier when they feel cared for. In this kind of positive environment, everyone flourishes. You will even start to look forward to your hectic days.

- ✓ Show them respect

These are people who are highly dependent on you. This makes it easy to disrespect them because there is nothing they can do about your bad attitude. However, disrespectful behavior is seen in shallow minded individuals and I believe you are not one of those. So, show compassion by being respectful to the people who need your care. The following examples describe how a respectful nurse ought to behave:

- Treat patients as equals: Remember, they are human, just as you are and their illness or suffering has not changed that fact.

- Respect their choices: You might be the caregiver and it's true that you know better. However, cease from imposing your unwanted ideas and opinions unless it is a matter of life and death. Respect their choices and wishes as much as possible and if you have to disagree, make sure you explain why—including when the patient is clearly not able to make good choices for themselves and you have to explain yourself to a next of kin.

- Knock on the door before entering their room. This act accords them respect, dignity, and privacy. Sure, it's 'your hospital' and they just borrowed the room, but it is their room for now. I'm sure you would be mad if anyone just bugged in your room when you could be crying or, worse, naked.

- Explain tests and procedures that they have to go through. You are the professional and you know what's best in their situation, but it is always good to have a patient understand clearly what's being done. It makes them feel important, respected and somewhat in control and not some guinea pig in a lab.

Compassion for Self

So far, we have looked at how we can show compassion towards those we serve. However, we are yet to discuss compassion for the person who matters the most here: you. If your wellbeing is compromised, no one will be happy and there is no healthcare. As you shower others with compassion, never forget you need it too.

According to research by the Centers of Disease Control, the nursing profession has been classified as one of the most stressful. The demands and nature of this job are not easy to deal with. We have mentioned it lots of times so far, but I will say it again: It is important that you remember that it will never be easy and these principles will help to help yourself, which will then help you to help others. This is for you as much as it is for them. As RuPaul said, "'If you don't love yourself, how in the hell you gonna love somebody else?"

My story of self-compassion, or lack there of

I am going to tell you about an experience in my career that taught me just how important it is to be kind to self and cut yourself some slack, despite your mess-ups. If it wasn't for self-compassion, I would not be celebrating 20+ years in the nursing profession today. I would probably be a front office assistant somewhere powdering my nose every ten minutes. Not that I have anything against front office assistants.

I had been a nurse for about 1 year but working in a hospital for about 6 months. I remember like it was yesterday. It was a Friday evening as I was working the night shift, one of those days when you wish you could be in your bed, snuggling with your dog, watching Netflix. Instead of resting during the day when I was off duty, I'd had to go home and attend to my sick mum. To cut the long story short, I will tell you that I was dead tired and was struggling to stay alert.

They say when it rains it pours. I was already feeling like crap and on this very same day, I made the worst medical error that made me feel worse. I was sad, embarrassed and I had never doubted my career choice until this day. I almost left my job, as I had written and handed in my resignation letter, convinced that I was this messed up individual who did not deserve to be trusted with people's health.

A middle-aged had man walked in. His legs were fine, but he was very drunk and could not carry him well. His left hand, though, was hanging loose at the elbow. It was a ghastly sight; a lot of blood trailed behind him.

One look at him and the nurses on duty ran. And I don't mean they all ran towards him. No, many fled towards other rooms where they were not needed, playing busy to avoid the medical 'disaster' that had just walked in. I won't say that I did not think of running to 'check on' patients; the thought crossed my mind, several times as I stared at him blankly. I could not just leave him there. I was a good nurse. Right?

It was obvious he needed surgery immediately or he would bleed to death. So, we—the few remaining nurses—we wheeled him to the emergency room. It would take a long time to explain how I ended up being the only one preparing him for the procedure, so I won't bother getting into it.

I did not know his weight, there was no time to check considering the heavy bleeding let alone the fact that he could not stand. So, I asked him, since he could talk. Amid the insults of a rotten drunk, I got his weight and there, I calculated the dosage for the anesthesia. Let's just say, the surgery went well but the recovery from it, not so much. I had given him an overdose and instead of numbness, he fell into a deep sleep, a coma.

How did I overdose him? Well, getting weight details from a drunk in pain is not the most exact science. He probably guessed the figure or remembered it from 10 years ago, I don't know; but I know I shouldn't have taken his word. Now lay a man, comatose, because of me. He could die, they told me, and I would be responsible for that.

After all my nights in prayer, the heavens must have had mercy on me. He recovered a few days later. I breathed a sigh of relief. They told me that such things happen, and it was just one of the big tests I would have to overcome in my career. Mistakes happen, a doctor who admitted to making even worse mistakes told me. I was relieved but...

Not a day went by without me feeling that I was just too dumb and incompetent to be a nurse. I was embarrassed and I lost all self- belief. I felt like my life was ruined. I did not know what to do and I spent most of my time sitting out on some benches in the large hospital compound. It was here that I penned a resignation letter, sure that I was not fit for the career. Yes, I had worked hard for it and in my heart, I knew that caring for people in this way was I wanted to spent my life doing. My mind, however, counted my blunders and told me I was not fit for the job. So, I quit.

Fast forward, I am still a nurse. I found another nursing job, which is why I'm celebrating 20 years in the career, and writing this book. How did I manage to get back after all that defeat, self-doubt, and criticism? I found something that the previous me didn't know after a year of nursing: Self-compassion.

In that light, let me tell you what I would tell my younger self and every other nurse feeling the same way because of mistakes they have made, or tough times faced.

Lessons on How to Be Compassionate to Self

No one ever promised you that it will always be easy, you will always get everything right, or that you would never make a nursing error. Trust me when I say mistakes, some life threatening, are bound to happen. You will mess up big time. However, does blaming yourself, quitting, feeling embarrassed, and beating yourself up ever change anything? I'm sure you have done it, so tell me, how much better did you feel?

I did not feel better after blaming myself and quitting. It only got worse and I was on the verge of breaking; I had gotten so miserable and was losing my mind—quite literally. I'm sure you blaming yourself didn't help you feel better either.

After I quit, people close by who knew I was a nurse wondered if I was on leave or something and why my previously beautiful hair was so messed up. The path of misery was not working out well for me. Fortunately, a dear friend showed me another path, of cutting myself some slack, as they called it. In other words, self- compassion. It helped to restore me to my career and myself.

Nurses go through a lot. If we lacked self-compassion, we would have hospitals full of nothing but self-hating maniacs. I'm sure you have seen some. They do not give a damn about themselves, or anyone for that matter. Woe unto you if you work with one.

It's worth it to learn to love yourself, imperfect as you are and as you will always be. Let's learn a few things about self-compassion, shall we?

Truths Versus Myths of Self-Compassion

Myth: Being compassionate to self means having self-pity

Truth: There is nothing pitiful with compassion.

Self-pity means drowning in your struggles and weaknesses and thinking that you are supposed to sit in a corner and cry. It's the mentality that the world is unfair to you, forgetting that everyone else is having it bad too, if not worse.

When you are being compassionate to self, you do not pretend that you aren't suffering with the 'I am fine' punch line. You admit the fact that you are suffering or struggling and realize that nobody is being unfair to you; other people have problems too. Also, you do not allow your mind to over think and blow your issues out of proportion. You see them for what they are; no additions or subtractions.

Like in my story above, overdosing a patient because I made a mistake about their weight was just that; an overdosing mistake – which anyone can make when they are tired and dealing with a freaking drunk. There was nothing about incompetence or dumbness in it – my over thinking mind made that up.

Myth: Self-compassion encourages slothfulness and irresponsibility

Truth: Being kind to self has nothing to do with being slothful or irresponsible.

Self-compassion means that you take responsibility for whatever is going on, understanding that fussing and beating yourself up about it will not do you or anyone else any good. So, you take the high road: You forgive yourself, you find a way to deal with it, learn from your mistakes. Then you let go of the hurt and move on.

Myth: You cannot move forward with self-compassion; self-criticism is the ultimate motivator.

Truth: Telling yourself how dumb you are over and over again does not motivate anyone.

If you ask me, being overly self-critical is fueling hate towards the person you ought to love the most: Yourself. If anything, you are inspiring yourself to mess up even more.

Consider this: Do you know how pre-Millennials were raised Parents used to be harsh; they thought punishment, mistreatment, and criticism would keep a child in line. For example, children were denied food for the most trivial mistake.

Today, society has matured beyond that primitivism (sorry, Mom) and learned that being supportive and encouraging is the best way to raise kids. We love them despite their imperfections. When they make a mistake, we do not chase them away or deny them food; instead, we address their mistakes, make them take responsibility and show them a better way to do things. All the while, we keep them close with love.

This is exactly how self-compassion works. We do not criticize; that is old fashioned. We accept our failures, accept ourselves (imperfections and all), learn from our mistakes and work on adopting healthy behaviors to replace those that cause us to screw up. You do not say, "I'm a failure." You say, "I failed at this, but I can try again," or "I should use another approach."

Practicing Self Compassion

Here are 5 ways to start practicing self-compassion and stop being such a bitch to yourself:

- Allow yourself to be imperfect

"Man is to err," goes a famous saying. The fact that you are human means that you will have flaws, you will never be perfect, and you will make mistakes. Lots of them.

We have grown up in a society where perfection is overrated. So, we think that imperfection is something terrible. Come on, now. You are not an angel, you are human. You should give yourself space to be so. Yes, make it okay to be flawed, lazy, sensitive, dumb, lost, you name it. Although the states of being that you do not think are admirable as part of your human nature, you should never define yourself by them. I mean, you can be sensitive and cry behind the curtain when a patient's suffering gets to you without letting it define you, or losing faith in your potential and ability to handle the situation. It is only human to feel that way, so cry and then step up your care for them. You may help them feel better if you do.

- Treat yourself as you would a little child

What would you tell a small child who had accidentally spilled ink on her beautiful drawing? "You are such a screw-up, can't you do anything right?" or, "It's okay. This is ruined, but I can help you make another one. And this time, we should keep the ink far away"? I bet you would choose the second statement. It would cheer them up. The first one will make them sad, give up or even worse. It will engrave in their mind that they are stupid as hell and mistakes mean you have reached a dead end.

So, if you picked the second statement to comfort a child, you must always pick similar approaches when it comes to yourself. Whenever you fear pain or when you fail, remember that little child and what you would do for them and then do it for yourself. Comforting and encouraging encourage yourself, don't keep emotions indefinitely bottled up, push yourself to try harder. Do it for you.

- Look at the bigger picture

During times of struggle or suffering, we tend to focus on the now and feel trapped. We try so hard to emotionally survive the present ugly moment, and this is where over-thinking, self-blame, and criticism comes in. Focusing on this moment makes it seem like the world is over, which is never the case.

The truth is, what's done is done, the moment will pass. People may talk about it but tomorrow or in a few days, there will be new things for them to think of and talk about. So, when you are feeling the pressure to be mad and hard on yourself in the moment, think about tomorrow, when all this will be behind you. Will there be any love left inside of you to take you through tomorrow? Only you can decide.

- Adopt a growth mindset

You should avoid the way of thinking that keeps you hellbent on things being a certain way. This way of thinking holds to the idea that things such as personal attributes like intelligence, knowledge and personality are carved in stone or rather they are in-born.

For instance, you are either intelligent or not or you have knowledge about something or you do not. This mindset creates a need for you to prove yourself to others and even yourself over and over again. You try your utmost not to 'look stupid'; any mistake has lethal effect on self-esteem as it proves where you lack in the 'top qualities'. You break when you face challenges of frustration and failure that just proves how stupid you are. This is called a fixed mindset.

On the other hand, a growth mindset is based on a belief that you can develop those basic qualities and 'top attributes'. Intelligence and knowledge is not static or inborn; it can be cultivated through effort. For people with the growth mindset, mistakes or failure are opportunities to learn and grow. This person believes that even though they may falter, they can learn to do anything they want and improve through application and exercise.

As you can see, the growth mindset will help you cope in this tough career. You are definitely going to face challenges, and it will help you bounce back when you feel like you should just pack up and go home. It will also keep the flame of self-love burning and shut down that self-critic bitch who tells you how you can't do this or that because you failed. The growth mindset tells you that you can learn how to do better, and that failure or mistakes are not a death sentence, but where the fun begins.

- Learn to forgive

In addition to accepting the fact that imperfection is part of the human experience, you should learn to practice forgiveness. Yes, forgive yourself when you mess up.

I know it's not an easy thing to do. Our minds are good at reminding us of our mistakes ever so often so we feel bad. That's okay, though; what matters is that you do not dwell on this emotion. Just allow it to surface. It will soon get tired and shrink away if you don't give it any attention.

Also, detach your sense of self-worth and self-love from performance or perfection. It removes the expectation that you have to be a certain way or achieve a certain thing to deserve your own love. This way, a mistake will just be a mistake and it will be easier to forgive and be gentle with yourself. As Melanie Koulouris says, "There is no sense in punishing your future for the mistakes of your past. Forgive yourself, grow from it, and then let it go."

- Practice mindfulness

Mindfulness helps you to be present and fully experience the present moment. In mindfulness, when something painful happens, you feel it, face it head on, and acknowledge it. It is not a pleasant experience, so it's no wonder many people like to skip this part and go straight to problem solving or blaming.

However, facing your pain and suffering as when you are in doubt, tired, or have messed up big time is way better than hiding from it. This is because facing through situations makes you more likely to accept, learn and move on. Hiding or running away from them make you hostage to them; you will always have that negative voice in the back of your mind reminding you of it. This is how people become depressed and hate themselves so much they want to die.

There is another reason why you have to be mindful: to be aware of and conquer your inner critic. Self-criticism has a way of creeping in and playing on repeat in our minds. When you are experiencing what is happening now, you are aware of the thoughts that are flowing. You are then able to arrest the negative and false self- defeating thoughts before they start playing on repeat and appearing to be true. By being aware of your thoughts, you are able to take charge and intentionally direct your mind to think positive, even when you are bombarded by negativity.

3: Patience

They say patience is a virtue, one that is important, but elusive. In the modern world where almost each one of our whims is satisfied with a click of a button, we have not learned patience.

What is Patience?

Some say that patience is the ability to wait. However, I believe that patience is the ability to tolerate waiting, frustration, or delay, with calmness. It is not easy to be patient, but it's worth it. Impatience is ridiculous and, to some degree, crazy. It is not worth it, not at all.

Consider the following situation:

It's evening. You are so damn tired from being on your feet attending to people all day. You pass by the convenient store to get some food supplies. There is a long queue at the cashier, and even worse, its moving at a snail pace. The cashier is taking their sweet time.

You get so angry you could explode. Such turmoil is going through your head and you are about ready to kill somebody. You just want to reach over and wring their neck. Your feet hurt and you afford to be cannot be standing there for half an hour. You're thinking they have no respect for the same persons who get them paid. How in the world could anyone be so slow? Why can't they do their job right? Arrrrgh!!

I can see a problem with the above type of thinking, can you? You see, all the above turmoil in your brain is not hurting anyone else more than it is hurting you. Yes, you may yell at the cashier and start a ruckus, leaving them anxious or something. However, the greatest effect is on you. It is your mind that is in turmoil; it is your body that stress hormones are tearing into; it's your nerves that are on edge, your heart that is pounding and racing, and your blood that is boiling. The only person who is getting really tortured is your pitiful self.

What's worse, the torture is all for nothing. You will still be stuck in that queue. Your impatience has not moved you to the front of the queue, in a traffic jam, at lunch with a friend who never stops talking about their ex-boyfriend, stuck with the patient who won't stop complaining, and so on.

Impatience is not helpful. Patience is the ultimate antidote.

Components of Patience

Patience speaks the language of:

Self-control: The ability to regulate your thoughts, emotions and behavior when you are faced with temptation (like the slow cashier, the rude lady, etc.) or an impulse. For instance, when you could be mad that the cashier is slow, you choose to think that maybe they had a long day and they are as tired as you.

Restraint: The ability to moderate one's behavior or reactions. For instance, when someone insults you, do not react badly, say, by hitting them or insulting them back. In other words, restraint is showing calm, sensible and controlled behavior when you could act in a volatile—even if understandable—manner.

Delayed gratification: The ability to give up what you could get now to wait to achieve a bigger goal in the future. The impulse for immediate reward tends to be quite strong. For instance, you could sacrifice sleep or dinner with a love interest to get a task finished so you can rest easy tomorrow or go for your friend's party.

The Importance of Patience in Nursing

You take on a lot of stress as a nurse, whether you work in a fast- paced hospital environment or just visiting the sick in their homes. The mere fact that you have to care of people in vulnerable situations makes it inevitable that you will run into difficult situations every now and then.

Given the nature of your work, you may have to sacrifice sleep on many occasions and still be expected to show up ready for action on the next shift. Other times, you may encounter a rude doctor who pushes you around, a complaining patient or an overbearing relative. It is not easy to take all this crap and maintain a level head.

Patience helps in any situation. It prevents you from getting worked up and losing your mind in this environment.

- It helps you to stay calm

When a patient is displaying challenging behavior or their relative is overreacting, patience enables you to step back and take a breath before you react. You can stomach the anger and frustration building within.

You might be feeling the need to give them a piece of your mind or chase them out of the facility but then you have the ability to tolerate the emotions and their annoying behavior without blowing up.

- You are better placed to think and act rationally

When you have a cool head on your shoulders, you are able to think clearly and act rationally. You agree with me that dealing with a stressful situation while stressed brings forth unpleasant outcomes. However, when you are calm, you have a more peaceful and reasonable approach. You do not look frustrated and out of line like the rest of them. Instead, you manage to calmly take control of the situation and patients see that.

- It helps your physiological wellness

By maintaining calm, our mental and physical health is greatly improved. I'm sure you will agree with me that, when you lose it, you feel a heaviness in your heart, limbs, and even your mind. This is just a feeling that we often shrug off as normal, but what we don't know is that this heaviness is taking a toll on our well-being. Sooner or later, there will be unexplainable migraines, backaches, hypertension, you name it.

Getting worked up triggers the release of stress hormone, which increases the heart rate, interferes with insulin, and raises blood pressure.

Essentially, impatience will mess with your body. You'd better calm the hell down. You need your health to be in top shake because your job is tough and poor health will impact it negatively.

- It helps you to maintain focus

If you have been worked up before (which I know you have), you know that it was difficult to maintain your focus on the task at hand. This is because the turmoil inside your body fogs up your brain, especially because you get anxious, stressed and frustrated.

Then your focus is all over the place.

Patience fosters mental calmness and clarity, which enables you to maintain your focus. This is a state which allows you to participate fully in every experience you have. You know how important this is in healthcare. You do not want to be making mistakes, now, do you?

- It helps strengthen your relationships with others

Patience—or the lack thereof—is notorious for creeping out through your non-verbal cues. This means that people can read impatience on you, and it sure is a turn off.

The environment you find yourself in as a nurse puts you in the middle of emotional and physically vulnerable people who are looking to you for help support. What happens if they read impatience on your face? It does not bring out the best in them, to say the least. They get anxious, stressed, and afraid to even ask for your help or advice.

Patience helps a caregiver develop understanding and compassion, all of which are important in strengthening relationships between colleagues as well as patients. You will be seen as supportive, kind and calm, and people are likely to be more open and cooperative with you. This is how good relationships are created.

- It helps create a healthy environment

You know how tension hangs in the air like thick fog in medical facilities. It's inevitable since no one comes there for a party; they are either sick themselves or they have a sick patient. So, imagine if you add impatient caregivers to that.

What would the hospital environment be like? Depressing as hell, don't you think?

A patient nurse is like seasoning for the 'meal' of the healthcare experience. They make a tense environment easier to bear as they exude hope. Patience puts people at ease and makes them feel like they are being heard and cared for.

Consider the following examples:

Being patient with an overbearing supervisor keeps tension and bad blood at bay. Even though you could give them a piece of your mind, you choose to tolerate them and be humble instead. If a patient is showing difficult behavior, patience helps you understand them and be compassionate so you do not reflect that behavior. Instead, you listen to all them, no matter how much bile they spew, and still manage to reassure them and give the care they need.

You agree with me that these kinds of good reactions, even when you are in challenging situations, kind of makes the air lighter and things better. It results in a healthy work environment.

There is just one more thing that patience can do for you; it can make you impact a life greatly. It could be someone else's life or even yours.

Patience Impacts Lives Positively: A Sweet Story of Patience

Once, I was doing my final rounds to check on my patients before my shift ended. It had been a long day and I was exhausted. I could not wait to get home to kick my shoes off, take off the pants that had started to feel like they were strangling my body, and stretch out on my couch. I was already daydreaming about it and I could barely focus on the patients.

"Nurse, please," called a small soft voice from behind. I was done checking the last room and was a few minutes out from getting out the hospital. I frowned, but I did not let them see it. I was hoping against hope that it was not someone who was going to delay me with some trivial issue.

I turned around with a smile (a plastic one), not really knowing who to face as I did not quite make out where the voice was coming from. A hand was raised right by the left corner of the room. I walked up to the bed where a young teenage girl, about 14 years of age lay. She had long jet-black hair and a round face with small squinted brown eyes. She was smiling when I said "Yes, please."

"I would like to go to the terrace," she said. "I want some air. Can you take me?"

That was just what I needed, someone delaying me on purpose.

She couldn't have picked a better time to bother me. And what air was up at the terrace? We had excellent air conditioning, there was enough air in the room!

I did not tell her all of that, of course. When I looked back at her, she was staring at me, as if she could read my face. I was embarrassed. Without a word, I helped her out of bed and held her as we walked to the terrace. (She refused to sit in a wheelchair.)

She seemed to have gotten another lease of life by getting that air she so yearned for. She was not squinting anymore, and I could now see that her eyes were quite big. Her smile was contagious; I could not help but smile, too, without even realizing why. She said I should smile more, to show off my dazzling smile.

That compliment broke the ice and got us talking. We moved from smiles and teeth to fashion then to childhood memories. I told her stories of my teenage years and we laughed about the crazy things I did to get the attention of my crush, a neighbor who had just moved to our neighborhood with his parents during my first year of high school. I had even 'kidnapped' their straying cat so he could come looking for it and at least talk to me.

She said my ways were old school and foolish and laughed her heart out as she shared her experiences in the current world and what she would have done if she were me. We sat there a long time and relived so many nostalgic memories.

Kimberly (that was her name) had this dreamy look in her eyes when she finally said she was getting cold and we needed to go back inside. Two hours had passed since my shift ended and another nurse had taken over. I had to hand over Kimberly to her, but the patient would not have it. She had me put her in bed. Gosh, she looked so fresh! I couldn't stop myself from giving her a bear hug and a kiss on the forehead. She was going to have a great night, she said. As I was turning to leave, she grasped my hand and pulled me down so she could whisper in my ear. She said, "Thank you for so much air, cat thief." I smiled, pulled her nose gently and left giggling. That night, I really had a great night to say the least. I got so much air along with Kimberly. I felt free.

I reported to work the next morning to find Kimberly's bed empty and her roommates sobbing. I thought she'd had another hemorrhage (she had a tumor in her brain that made her bleed through the nose and ears) and was at the emergency room. It would not be the first time since her operation. So, I rushed there but I did not find her. I learnt from the night shift nurse that Kimberly had succumbed to her illness and passed on peacefully in her sleep, holding her pink bear.

Gosh! That girl had suffered so much but she had looked so healthy when I left. That's when it hit me: she was just acting strong. She somehow felt that she was losing the fight and she wanted to spend the last moments celebrating her life, as short as it had been. All those stories she had told me, she just wanted to relive it one last time. She needed someone to share with and she chose me. But why?

I went to the terrace and let the tears flow as I sat exactly where she had sat. I was sad but at the same time, I felt glad I had been there for her, even though I had not wanted to at first. I am thankful I chose to be patient. Imagine if she had met an angry nurse, impatient to end their shift and go home. How would she have lived her last moments? I hate to think of it. Kimberly did rest forever, with so much air and laughter. I am glad I gave her that. So far, I don't think I have done anything more important in my career.

That event changed my life and my approach to situations. I appreciate the little joys and small moments and I am a lot more patient. I am happier and a better person since I now look at life from a different, more patient perspective. I am not in a hurry to experience life.

Thank you, Kimberly...

How to Cultivate Patience

You may think that you were born impatient, that you cannot tolerate a wait or frustration and you have to say or do what comes to your mind to get relief. In the streets, they call it keeping it real. I call it immaturity and stupidity.

The 'keeping it real' that makes you act in the heat of the moment will cause you to hurt people, your career and yourself. It is a vice you have learned and which you can unlearn.

Patience is neither inborn nor inherited. It is true that some of us are naturally built to be more tolerant, but it is important to understand that the virtue is a skill which can be learned by anyone who is willing to put in the work.

The following strategies are the best for learning the virtue of patience:

- **Beware and be mindful of your triggers**

You do not just become impatient; there is always a reason behind it, a trigger. It could be people who look or behave in a certain way, situations or just phrases. For instance, my boss loses his patience when people say, “That’s not possible,” and I cannot stand people with ‘know it all’ attitude; I just lose it.

How to find your triggers

There are a few things that cause you to enter an impatient state of mind. You should identify them and probably write them down.

- Think about it

Take some time to think about the last time you lost your cool. What caused it? Think of why you reacted that way and write it down.

P.S.: You are talking to yourself, so do not make up the excuses and stories you tell others to try to look justified in your actions. What’s the real reason why you lost it?

- Ask people around you

Since we act with impatience unconsciously, you might not know all your triggers. In this case, you should ask your friends and co- workers about it. They could know a few things that 'set you off,' which you do not have a conscious knowledge of.

- Check your body

I find that I lose my cool easily when I am hungry or tired. Yes, that's me. How about you?

The truth is; many people's impatience is fueled by physical factors affecting the body. They include hunger, fatigue, dehydration or pain (such as a headache). Have you ever noticed that you start your workday willing to help and to go the extra mile, but a few hours into it, you start going off at the slightest provocation? This explains it.

So, the next time you feel impatient, check your body. Close your eyes, force yourself to calm down and do a body scan. Shut out the noise from outside and tune into what your body is communicating. You may just need a meal or a rest.

- Keep a 'patience' journal

Have a journal, call it the 'patience' journal. In this journal, record every instance you start to feel impatient. Make sure to write down what the situation is and why it is making you feel so frustrated. Of course, you may not be able to jot it down at the actual moment since you could be attending to people at work.

However, you can make a mental note (it counts, too) and transfer it later or scribble on a piece of paper next to you, as if you were writing something important. Notice that this, too, gives you a moment to pause and breathe. By writing down, you keep a track of your impatient moments and their causes. This way, you will identify the recurrent culprits.

Why is identifying your triggers important?

- It makes you aware of your reactions and reasons behind it. With this awareness, you are more likely to catch yourself before you go over the edge of impatience and make a better choice. For instance, if its hunger, you know how it gets you so you will leave your post (before you start yelling at people) and have a snack.

- You are in a better place to devise successful strategies to avoid being impatient.
- Intentionally make yourself wait

They say practice makes perfect. It works in every area of your life, even in learning the skill of patience. Maybe you lack it because you have taught yourself to get what you want when you want it; instant gratification. The only way you teach yourself to wait is by practicing it. You do not have to wait for anything grand like marriage or falling in love; it works when you start with the small, seemingly insignificant areas of your life.

Do you feel like watching the new season of your favorite show on Tuesday? Put it off until the weekend and find something productive to fill the time before then; you know, to occupy the mind and minimize temptation. Do you want to grab the chocolate bar on your bedside table the moment you step out of bed? Make yourself wait for an hour and go have a glass of warm water first. If you really feel your fingers itch to open Instagram on your phone, wait it out for an hour. Did your little boy mess up the room you just arranged? Wait 30 minutes before you scold him and don't even look at the room.

When you practice this in your small tasks every day, you are strengthening the muscle of patience. Also, you will be wearing off that instant gratification bug. Soon, you will realize that it's not as urgent or as irritating as it seemed. I am certain that you will love the calm approach to stuff. It is from this small practice that you will spread 'the wait approach' to other irritating areas of your life.

- **Learn to embrace discomfort; be comfortable in the uncomfortable**

This is not a call to keep your hand over a flame when it is burning through your skin. It is a call to drop the belief that being comfortable is the only state we are entitled to and the one state we can tolerate. This is because life with its unpredictability will often throw you curves, big and small, good and bad. Often, you will be thrown out of your comfort zone, and you get impatient with the circumstances, desperate for the comfortable space we are used to.

When you desire the comfortable but still have room to accept and tolerate the uncomfortable, you are more likely to be patient. Best believe that most things, especially those that benefit you later, will not feel as good as you want them to. A good example is when you want to stop drinking large amounts of caffeine to be alert and instead drink enough water. Think of the side effects of caffeine withdrawal; it is not going to feel great, is it? But, it's for the best.

What do you do when you want to flee from the uncomfortable? Say, "This is just uncomfortable, not intolerable," and stay the course. It will help build your tolerance and, more importantly, your patience, to be applied in other more distressing areas. For example, when a colleague calls to say they will be late and you have to extend your shift to cover for them. It is uncomfortable but not intolerable.

How to Manage Impatience

It is inevitable that we will get impatient every now and then, especially in our line of work. We are likely to meet annoying people and get in annoying situations; it can get ugly. It is easy to find yourself slipping into the vice of impatience. When that happens, here's how you can manage the situation:

- Pause, take a breath

Did you know that shallow breathing is a major sign of impatience and annoyance? So, stop and take a deep breath. When all else fails, this is a simple exercise, but it works. It can be done anywhere, even in front of your boss or client. They will think you are thinking of a response or just quiet because you have nothing to say in your defense but what they do not know is you are calming a rearing bear inside.

Breathing has the power to calm the mind and body; it slows down your quickening heart rate and relaxes your tense muscles. It helps ease the jitters and calm the turmoil building up in your mind that may come when things get annoying, complicated, and uncomfortable. So, take deep breaths. It may also help to count (inwardly) to ten before you speak.

- Act patient

Sometimes you will not feel so patient. Things may get so upsetting that you want to slap someone. In this case, act patient. Yes, you may not feel like it, but who said you have to feel like it all the time?

If you have to, force yourself to slow down, bite your lip, squeeze your hand, and hold a pen so tight it would break. Keep a straight face and, if possible, a (fake, yes) smile. It will appear to others that you are calm, even though you are not. You will find that, by acting patient, you start to feel more patient. You welcome patience back and chase out that ingrate impatience.

- Talk yourself out of it

Discourage yourself from being impatient by facing the truth that it does not get you anywhere. You have seen that it does not cause others to move faster or make things any better. If anything, it just makes the situation worse by stressing you and everyone out.

4: Empathy

What is Empathy?

A person is being empathetic if they can have the experience of understanding another's thoughts, emotions, their condition or situation from his or her point of view rather than one's own. This is to say they can put themselves in the other person's shoes and experience their situation as if it was their own.

Have you heard about emotional intelligence (EI), the state of being aware of your emotions and those of others? Well, empathy is a big part of EI. It creates the link between our own emotions and those of others. It is how we as human beings get to understand what others are feeling. This way, we are likely to be a little more understanding, compassionate and considerate and less mean.

Is Empathy The Same as Sympathy or Compassion?

Empathy, sympathy, and compassion are very often confused for good reason. All refer to relating to other's feelings, however they are very different in the way they are expressed and applied.

Compassion is closely related to empathy, except that the later involves feeling others' emotions, as if it were yours. Compassion is more about understanding that they are feeling pain and wanting to help. In other words, compassion works together with empathy. We already got compassion covered; now let's get to sympathy and empathy.

Sympathy is more of understanding and acknowledgement of what someone is going through and feeling for them. In other words, you feel bad for them. You can imagine their pain, but you do not feel it or try to understand how it feels. It is associated with pity and sorrow for what another person is going through. But you leave it at that; just feeling bad for them but not getting intellectually or emotionally involved.

Empathy, on the other hand, engages the emotions in a more intimate way. It involves feeling with someone using your imagination.

Imagine you and a friend apply for the same job. You happen to get it, but they are rejected. If you are being sympathetic, you will feel bad for them. You will probably will say, "I am so sorry they did not pick you," and actually mean it. Being empathetic, however, means you feel the disappointment with them, as if it were you who was rejected.

To get a better understanding of empathy, we can think about actors and the characters they play. They are given a character description, their experiences, their personalities, and so on. They have to get to know that character and mimic them; they have to feel exactly what that character would feel and do what they would do in a certain situation through imagination. In the film industry, they call it 'owning the character.'

This is how Taraji P. Henson, a good levelheaded lady, is able to play with the crazy Cookie in Fox TV's Empire. You wouldn't think they are different people with very different personalities. I mean, I have seen Taraji off the show and she's nothing like Cookie. She imagines the character and walks in her shoes.

Now back to our example; in the described situation, you would be feeling the hurt with them, identifying with how they feels and doing what you would have loved another person to do for you if you were to find yourself in a similar situation. For instance, you may offer to help them find another opportunity elsewhere and share what you did different to hook the job.

Let me show you a real-life example of how different empathy and sympathy are in the results of a real-life situation:

Once, a friend and I went for interviews for the same job. I went first, armed with all the knowledge there was about nursing in preparation. My friend and I had revised everything the previous night. In the interview room, they did not ask me that. Instead, I was bombarded with silly questions.

I recall being asked why I was not married yet. The first thought was to tell them, “Are you my mother? Mind your goddamn business!” Instead, I cooked up a story of how boyfriends somehow found me unfit because I would not come over and clean for them. They found it quite funny and laughed openly at me. The interview then turned into a relationship story session. I don’t remember any serious conversation flowing after that.

I think they asked the same question to her and, knowing how much she hates it since she has a relative who brings it up all the time, I can guess her response was a ‘back off bitch’ kind of answer. Turns out it was a personality, temperament, and patience test. I passed, she failed.

As we talked about her rejected situation (because I wanted her to feel better), I shared this information and she realized her blunder. She later applied again and got the job at the same place. She had dropped her rotten attitude this time. If I wasn't for empathy, I would have just felt sorry for her, told her how sorry I was, and reported to work leaving her a destitute, jobless, and desperate graduate for one more year.

Well, I tell a lot of stories. What can I say? My life has been amusing. But I hope you now understand the difference between sympathy and the golden empathy? The point is, empathy is the most attractive and noble skill compared to sympathy. It is okay to feel sympathy, but empathy allows you to 'walk a mile' in another person's shoes, and it makes sure you help.

3 Types of Empathy

As you move from feeling with the other person to doing something to help the situation, you will undergo three types of empathy:

i. Cognitive empathy: When you are able to understand or connect with what the other person might be thinking. This puts you in a better position to communicate with them, as it helps you deliver information in a way that the other person will resonate with.

ii. Emotional empathy: When you are able to share in and relate to the feelings of the other person. It has been called the 'your pain in my heart' feeling. It will help you build an emotional connection with people.

iii. Compassionate empathy: This one goes deeper than just understanding and sharing in other people's feelings. However, it is driven by those abilities. It is the type of empathy that moves you to take action and assist where you can.

How These Branches of Empathy Work Together

Imagine that a colleague just lost their job because they made a simple mistake and your boss chose not to hear them out.

The natural reaction that anyone would have (except the evil person in the corner thinking, Good riddance, b**ch!) is sympathy. It may move you to say, "I am so sorry this happened to you. I hope you get another opportunity soon." Your friend may appreciate these words, but you will not have really helped them. You will dish the words and move on with your world, lest you get fired too.

However, empathy will take more effort, and it will actually help the other person. It starts with cognitive empathy. In this situation, you will imagine what your friend is going through, the kinds of questions in their heads. How am I going to pay my rent? How will I be able to get another job to send my kids are to school? How can I plead my case and get my job back? Who is going to defend me? This is unfair!

Emotional empathy will help you not only understand their pain but also share in it. You may not cry like they are, but you will definitely feel the hurt in your heart. You try to connect with something deep inside of you that knows this kind of pain. It may remind you of an event that sparked such feelings.

Compassionate empathy will finally set in as you relate to the other person's pain as if it were your own. Since you would not like anyone to go through such kind of pain, you are moved to do something about the situation. In this case, you might not be able to give their job back or convince your boss to hear them out but you can offer to help. You could share a few contacts that could help them find a new job, or offer to let their kids live with you for a while in a case where they are worried about being kicked out of the house or not being able to pay the sitter. Maybe you could just offer a simple, "You can count on me to help with anything that I can. Call me if you need anything, even if to talk."

Empathy in Healthcare: Clinical Empathy

When dealing with patients, we need to have clinical empathy, especially when you are relating with patients. It is a bit of detached kind of understanding. The Society for General Internal Medicine describes it as, "The act of correctly acknowledging the emotional state of another without experiencing that state oneself. This is very important, especially when it comes to maintaining a stable and friendly work environment. It is 'detached' because you avoid suffering personally along with people you are attending to. Otherwise, who would care for them?

As an aside, it should be noted that clinical empathy need not be applied to colleagues.

The Significance of Empathy in Nursing

- It makes a whole lot of difference to the nature and quality of care

Empathy is very crucial in healthcare. It is important that a caregiver can relate to the experience of their patients and be moved to help. You see, when we look at healthcare from the perspective of the patient, it is centered on difficult situations and emotions. Being sick is hard, both physically and emotionally.

You will find that even in the 'happy' healthcare situations like having a baby, emotions are riding high and usually darker emotions such as fear and stress are ever-present. A patient needs a person who cares enough to understand what they are going through and who can do everything to ease their suffering.

There is also the issue of healthcare literacy. In today's system, 'fake news' in healthcare has become a major problem. They come from misinformation – those misinformed stories we get from people out there; medics and cab drives, alike. Fake news gets patients confused and most times overwhelmed by fear, anxiety and stress. You can imagine going to a hospital with a certain condition and people telling you false stories about your condition.

I remember a patient who came in with a rather serious injury on their knee. Before I could even attend to them, he said, “We are cutting it off. Get me the papers I need to sign.”

Why the hell would anyone want to cut off their leg? As I found out later, he had been told that the knee is very sensitive and such injuries never healed; that he would be receiving treatment for a very long time, perhaps the rest of his life. This is why this guy was ready to let the leg go rather than be in and out of hospital the rest of his life. From the look on his face and his tone, he had already made peace with cutting it off.

With some quiver in his voice, I asked, “Are you sure?” It was this that caused me to dig deeper and find out the information he had about his condition. This is how fake news nearly cost someone their leg if he had met someone who did not give any flying farts.

So, it should be quite evident that empathy will and does make a huge difference in healthcare.

Benefits of Clinical Empathy

Sympathy is easy and 'enough' to get you through any medical issue, but empathy matters.

- It is the number one patient satisfaction tool

You may give them medication, good clothing and a nice environment but, without empathetic care, all those other measures are quite useless.

Patients want a person they can easily relate to; a person who shows them that they understand their situation, their feelings and their perspective. They want to feel a connection and experience trust and comfort with their caregivers. Any person in pain or distress would want this, as it makes them feel that they are actually being cared for.

- It improves patients' outcomes

A person who lived healthy life developed an infection and has an enormous wound on their leg. They need crutches to help them walk. It is a big life change, the type of change people struggle to accept and live with.

Do you think that a perfectly changed dressing on the wound gives the patient the will to live and cope with their new struggle? Yes, it will keep the wound clean and uninfected, reducing pain, but this is physical. How about the emotional wound? That needs addressing, too.

By taking the time to talk to them, encouraging them and listening to them talk about their fears or worries, reassuring them, explaining medical processes, or addressing any queries they may have, you are making them feel valued, respected and understood. Also, by engaging with them, you are helping heal that inner wound, which is beyond the reach of medical prescriptions. As a result, there are better patient outcomes: happier, satisfied, emotionally and physically well patients at the end of the day.

- It improves communication

By engaging with patients, better relationships are formed between them and their caregivers. As a result, there is better communication, understanding and trust. This offers a chance for proper guidance to them and empowerment of patients, which increases the effectiveness of treatment.

Common Empathy Mistakes

Sometimes you may not know what to say or do to make someone in a tough and painful situation feel better, even as a nurse. Other times, you may be too anxious or too sensitive yourself to offer a shoulder to lean on. Whatever you do, you should avoid committing the following empathy mistakes. In these situations, it may be better to excuse yourself from the patient. Yes, it may seem like you are offering help or comfort, but you're likely to make the situation worse if do the following:

- Pointing to the silver lining

Have you ever been telling someone a sad story of yours and before you are even done venting, they come up with this positive rubbish about the situation, telling you to look on the positive side? It did not feel good, did it? It feels like the person is not really hearing you or resonating with your pain. They seem to be avoiding your sad story, looking for something positive to talk about instead.

Statements such as "At least you did not die," "You should be grateful you have one good eye," "At least you can still conceive again," and "Everything happens for a reason" sound okay, but they are not really sensitive to a person's pain. They sugarcoat the pain and make them feel no better.

- Becoming an advisor

Being a nurse, you might be carried away by giving advice instead of giving a listening ear. Don't get me wrong; patients may appreciate your advice if the situation calls for it, and it could be helpful. However, in challenging times, that's not what people need unless ask for it. Sometimes, what a person who is suffering needs is not someone to add to the endless torrent of unsolicited advice. When they open up about their struggles, maybe all they need is someone to be there for them and just listen.

- Storytelling

You might think that narrating stories of someone else who went through a similar situation would help, but you're wrong. It beats all sense to think that a statement like, "Oh, I know someone who went through that. This is what happened..." would be beneficial. This is definitely not empathy. It appears as if you are just looking for something to divert attention from the sad story.

- Minimizing

A person struggling with a situation tells you about their pain and you go, "That's such a little problem. You will get over it, you'll see." Sounds encouraging, right?

However, the fact that you believe that they are strong enough to get through it does not mean that it isn't hard or it's not taking a toll on them. Statements like that minimize another person's pain and make them look like they are overplaying it by admitting that they are suffering. This is not helpful.

How To Use Empathy Effectively As A Caregiver

- Listen with all senses

Listen! Yes, learn to listen to the other person without interruptions or distractions. Listen to the entire message that the other person is trying to convey. Remember you are trying to 'get' this person, which is impossible if you have divided attention.

So, listen empathetically:

- ✓ Listen with your ears: hear the words being said and also take note of the tone of voice.

- ✓ Listen with your eyes: watch how they move their body as they speak. Most are the times people communicate more without saying a word.
- ✓ Listen with your heart: let your heart listen to their heart. What I mean is, try to listen to what they are feeling.
- ✓ Listen with your instincts: For example, do you sense that they are not communicating or they are leaving out something important?

- Put aside your viewpoint and try to see things from theirs

You have your viewpoint and it may not be similar to the other person's. Maybe yours is right. Nevertheless, put it aside and try to see things 'with their eye'. This helps you better understand where they are coming from and discourages judging and criticism.

When you try to see things as they do, you may realize that they are not evil, dramatic, stubborn or unreasonable as you may have presumed. You may come to realize that they are simply reacting from the knowledge they have or the capacity they are in.

- Acknowledge their perspective

When you can 'see' why people do what they do or hold certain beliefs, acknowledge their perspective instead of contesting it. This makes them feel appreciated and important, like they have a voice.

This does not mean that you have to agree with it; acknowledgement is not the same as agreement. It means that you may stick with your perspective but be open to the fact that people have different opinions. As they say, everyone is entitled to their own opinion. Acknowledging another person's perspective is simply a way of respecting their opinion.

- Develop others; have an orientation to serve

This involves taking action. It means that you act on the needs and concerns of the person in need. For instance, if they have been victims of 'fake news,' you are supposed to provide them with the correct information and make sure you deliver it in a language they would understand. This is what we call development.

Service orientation means that you put the needs of others before your own and seeking ways to improve their satisfaction or their experience. It means you can extend your shift by 10 minutes if a patient needs to share something with you. It means you can miss your lunch break to comfort a teenage girl whose illness is causing her to lose hope. In other words, it is selflessness in service.

When Empathy Is Hard And Overwhelming And How To Pull Through

It can be hard to be an empathetic caregiver. In your line of work, you are exposed to people who are not in the best state. It is easy to build a wall around yourself so that you do not get affected by their emotional states. Most caregivers would prefer sympathy; a simple 'I hope you feel better' or some other shallow words of comfort when a patient is crying about losing their child at birth and you walk way, never getting emotionally or intellectually involved to understand their situation. This is easier on our emotional being.

In my career, I have been guilty choosing sympathy because I wanted to protect myself. But, as we have discussed, empathy is best. However, protecting yourself from getting weighed down by all these emotions is important. You have a job to do; a job that requires you take care of people. You will need empathy in every case. Being an empathetic caregiver is like helping out someone in a hole by getting inside it first. It is okay to get in their hole, but it is crucial to get out very fast before you get stuck there too. If you cannot come out, then who will help them either of you? And remember there is another patient in another hole, waiting in the next room.

It can get overwhelming but you cannot afford to get an emotional overload. However, building a wall between you and the patients will not help the situation. You will have left them out in the cold. There are better ways to protect yourself from emotional overload.

If you feel it is happening to you, the following tips should help:

- Set emotional boundaries, not walls

You have to remain empathetic without becoming overly involved. So, you do not build walls – they completely block out people and turn you to a cold person. Boundaries, however, allow people in but only so far. Thus, you are protected while still being warmhearted.

The most successful way to set this boundary is by first finding yourself and connecting with your inner being. This way, you know what's yours and what's not and you have a clear vision of where others end and you begin.

To find yourself, you need self-awareness practices such as practicing mindfulness and meditation. A meditation yoga class would be fun. Find are calming practices for your body and mind calming that allow you to get grounded in yourself as you sit with the pain and suffering and bring presence to it. It is harmful to pretend such heavy feelings do not exist. It is by bringing them to the forefront that you are able to see them for what they are: absorbed, not yours. You can let them go, paving way for your own emotions to prevail.

- Be compassionate to self

When you give yourself enough compassion, you get to have enough emotional stability to be there for others. You need to take care of yourself maybe more than you care for others – and it does not mean that you become selfish. It means that you practice kind acts towards yourself.

We have discussed some of these acts earlier as we talked about self-compassion. They include taking some time off when you feel overwhelmed, positive self-talking, and engaging in activities that help you blow off some steam.

- Relieve yourself of emotional overload

Nurses are on the receiving end of some of the most awful situations, behaviors, and situations you can think of. The emotions they experience as a result are not pretty at all. They get what we call emotional overload or compassion fatigue, which can affect your health negatively.

So, since you cannot avoid emotional overload as you practice clinical empathy in your line of work, find a way to let those emotions out. The following tips should help.

- ✓ Build/find a support network

Talk about your emotions and what you go or went through with someone who would understand without judging or giving backlash. It could be your colleague, a member of a nurses' network (trust me, there is no better way to vent than sharing frustrations and concerns with someone who can relate), or maybe a close friend or spouse. Having an honest talk (the kind of talk without filters and you can say openly how a patient's odor disgusted you) will help you let out and let go, to refresh your emotions.

- ✓ Find an area in nursing that you are passionate about

Which specialty of nursing are you passionate about? Personally, I loved to work with kids, specializing in their mental health. I found this quite interesting and intriguing; I would wake up every day looking forward to work.

What do you want to specialize in? Find out and go serve in it. Once you do, you will find that no matter how hard your days are, you will be glad to report to the same job every single day and give your best.

5: Integrity

Integrity is a word that is thrown around a lot, maybe because it's a hot word for job application letters. However, not many people know what this word means or the kind of weight it bears. It's not a word that people give a lot of thought.

Today I want us to really give it thought. It is a very important component for every career, but it is extra important when it comes to careers for caring for people in vulnerable states, more so nursing.

If you were to define it, what would you say it is?

The Definition of Integrity

There are many possible ways to define integrity, but I would like us to take note of some keywords often missed in other definitions: Consistency, truthfulness, honesty, and accuracy of one's actions. They define the basic attributes of integrity.

Attributes of Integrity

- Consistency: This means that you remain the same regardless of the situation. For instance, you do not change according to your mood, environment or the persons around you. It means that if you are nice or compassionate, you will make a conscious choice to remain so in your next conversation or situation, even if you just had a fight with your spouse or friend.

- Honesty/accuracy of one's actions – this refers to authenticity of one's behavior, words and actions. It means that you mean what you say; you do not preach water and take wine (pun intended). Have you seen people who boast of certain values but when you look closely at their behavior, they do not uphold any of those values? For instance, I have a friend who says they value other people's opinions; that they are all for equality. It's true, they care about equality but are lacking in integrity. Why do I say that? It is because their behavior does not match their values. They will voice an opinion and shoot down any other that tries to compete with theirs.

In other words, when you have integrity, you have an inner sense of wholeness, honesty and a consistency of character. It should be seen in your words, actions, decisions, outcomes and behavior. You are the authentic you wherever you go, and don't wear masks depending on where you are and who you're with. If you are patient, there will not be an impatient you when you are tired. Also, there will not be a 'work you', 'home you', 'church you' or any other you.

You must have realized that integrity is not the simple thing people think it is. They say integrity is just being honest, but we now see that it is much more than just honesty.

We recognize that it can be extremely difficult to have integrity all the time. We are human and sometimes emotions get in the way. As a result, we are unable to manage our behaviors and actions and we cannot be our authentic selves because we are worried about others' opinion.

However, as hard as it is, living with integrity is the most important choice you can make for yourself, for people around you, and for those you serve.

Why Integrity is Important

- It earns you trust and respect, and helps create better relationships

If you have had someone betray you, then you know how much trust matters. It could have been a dear friend lying to you about something important, maybe even in an attempt to protect you from getting hurt. Their betrayal may have had an explanation, but could you get to trust them as much ever again?

Integrity demands that a person does the right thing, even (especially) when it is too damn hard to do so. In our example above, if your friend applied integrity, they would tell you what they have to, even if it would hurt you because they realize that it's the best thing to do. You are likely to get over the hurt feelings, but you will never forget that they risked your friendship to tell you what you needed to hear about a situation you cared about. I was once in a situation such as this:

Betrayal of a friend in the name of protection

Back when I was in high school, I had caught the 'fever' of wanting a smooth, even-toned face. So, I started using a new face cream and applied it two times a day religiously. I had a close friend, a roommate who watched me do it all. I asked them for an opinion of how my face was doing and they said it was fantastic.

I got some pimples and a teacher commented about my 'bleached' skin. Still, I asked my friend, and they told me not to listen to those 'naysayers.' Couple of weeks later, I got one of the worst acne breakouts I have ever suffered. Then, when we went on summer break, I had to explain to my parents why I was trying to bleach my skin. They even took me to psychologist.

Damn! My friend had been lying to me. I had not noticed my skin looking bleached, but everyone else could see it. When I called, furious, to ask why they did not tell me the truth, they said they were trying to protect me, so I would not feel bad. To make a long story short, I discarded everything that had gotten me to that point; the cream and my trusted friend.

This is exactly how lack of integrity works. But, with integrity, people get to trust and respect you, even if they cannot bear your blunt opinions. They respect and trust those who live with high morals and those who mean exactly what they say. At least they have confidence that you will always tell the truth, even if they do not like you. You see, nothing beats honesty; the worst truth is better than the worst lie.

- It makes you a great leader and earns you loyal followers

A good leader is not one who is right all the time. If you were to choose between a leader who charms everyone but never follows through on their promises and one who admits to not knowing it all but never breaks a promise, which one would you pick?

As a nurse, you are a leader. Great leadership in any field involves honesty. One who leads in integrity can admit that they are not perfect, and they do not have all the answers, but they work hard to achieve their goals or fulfill what they said they would.

This is what gets people to be loyal to them and to hang on their every word; they know they won't be let down. Integrity causes people to have unwavering faith in you, which is a very important factor in health care.

- It sustains the moral fabric of our society

In a society where our moral fabric is rotting with most people chasing after self-interests and gratification, we need people who believe in doing the right thing, even when there is no one to take a photo, give credit, or to fear.

For instance, a person who walks in integrity would not squander funds intended to help a certain group of people in need. They will give equal services to everyone and not prefer those who can part with a dollar or two. Corruption would be nonexistent. This integrity can do.

- It precedes you; it describes you before you can speak of your character

Integrity defines your character, which speaks so loudly people cannot hear what you are saying (who you claim to be). Your moral standing dictate what you do, and this alone tells people who you are. It can tell people that you are a person worth their trust, if they can count on you, and whether they should associate themselves with you or not. It does not matter what you say; your integrity (or lack thereof) precedes you

Importance of Integrity in the Nursing World

- It helps build trust among health care workers and between patients and the health workers

Integrity in healthcare encompasses the values of honesty, keeping one's word and adhering to codes of ethics, regardless of the situation or circumstance they find themselves in. A physician's or nurse's integrity helps build trust among healthcare professionals and between them and patients.

A doctor should be able to trust that the nurse taking care of his patients will follow instructions and do what's best for their wellbeing in any situation. Likewise, the patient should be able to put their trust in the physician or nurse handling them because their life is quite literally in their hands.

- It helps with moral dilemmas

In nursing practice, facing moral dilemmas is part of the job. We handle moral distress all the time in dealing with pain, suffering, and life and death.

A good example is a mother who chooses to put her wellbeing on the line to ensure that her unborn baby, who is very small baby and has a slim chance of survival, takes a breath of life. You have to support their decision by making sure this baby lives. It may require a lot of painful and dangerous procedures and they are aware that the baby may be suffering, and they may suffer mental or physical incapacities in future as a result.

Other times, we may find ourselves dealing with a patient who just attempted suicide and somehow came out alive, but dancing very close to the edge. They made a decision, a terrible one and landed in our care and now we are tasked with making sure that they pull through, even if it's not certain that they will.

These are situations that put a nurse in distress and make them face moral dilemmas. As in the cases above, they could be struggling with bringing themselves to follow all orders of treatment. In the first case, they wonder if they should allow such a young soul go through all that pain with a probability of coming out with lifelong health problems. In the second case, a nurse must spend long hours giving intensive care to save the life of a person who tried to end it.

It is in cases like these (and others like deciding which patient to attend to first; following the order of booking or attending to the yelling one first) that integrity helps a nurse make the right decision.

In my nursing career, I have witnessed nurses being asked to perform procedures that are completely unethical and which are considered immoral in nursing. Either they do it or compromise their job. I have seen patients from high social classes come in on their high horses expecting to be given special treatment and turned down. I have also known nurses who have preferred to be sacked than compromise what they believe to be right.

Integrity is Personal

Nursing is a profession which depends on one's principles and moral standing. Yes, there is a code of ethics and set morals to follow, but without a high moral standing and your own ethics to follow, there would be a problem. You see, nursing is more than following orders. A nurse should be able to carry out their duties in by aligning with their own values, integrity, and moral courage.

For the best outcomes, integrity is a very important attribute. At the very least it gives a guarantee that you will make an ethically correct decision when faced with moral dilemmas or when under distress. A doctor, a patient, and their family should be able to trust that you will do the right thing, even if the person you are tasked with is in a vegetative state and cannot see or report your actions.

Working in integrity, you will guide the suicide attempt victim through to better health and frame of mind without wondering why you should go through the trouble when you could let the patient have what they were seeking. Also, you will give equal treatment to all, without favorites or preferences.

Building Your Integrity

We may have gone through stuff or developed habits that have made our integrity weak. For instance, you could be talking too much and making promises you cannot keep, even to yourself. Also, you may have grown to prefer the road of least resistance, making you a person who prefers unethical shortcuts and compromises to having to go the long, hard way. You can build your integrity to correct your character flaws and improve your relationships by building trust and earning respect (even with yourself; there is a lot at stake if you cannot trust yourself to do the right thing).

It will take time, I guarantee it. You will have to start with honing the little areas of your life as person and as a nurse to develop integrity.

Tips for building your integrity from the ground up

- Be bluntly honest with yourself

We tell lies to people, but none are as deadly as the ones we tell ourselves (if you do not agree with this, you just confirmed its true). Try something different; stop the lies, the excuses and justifications.

Learn to question your actions. Not only that; question also your motives. Deep down, what's the reason behind your actions? You see, sometimes we do good things but with wrong motives. For instance, you may attend to someone well, not because it's the right thing to do, but because you want some token of appreciation, even just to be recognized by an onlooker.

Stop excusing your misdeeds. Instead of justifying what you know is wrong, learn to own up to your mistakes and then seek to do better. What I mean is: correct yourself and do not entertain your doing stuff that you are not proud of. As they say, charity begins at home, so integrity begins with you. Be honest, truthful, trustworthy with yourself, then it can spread to the rest of the world.

- Live a transparent life

Live transparently. This is not to say that you should hang your life on the skyline for everyone to see. It means that you should live your authentic life every single day; you should never pretend to be someone you are not. If you are true to yourself first, every other area of your life falls into an honest place.

It is normal to feel that you have to hide your shortcomings so that people do not think less of you. As a result, we create an illusion of a life that we would like to have but which we do not have. We know that this causes you to lie about things, and you know how one lie develops into a string of lies. If you want to live with integrity, you must avoid those little white lies and live transparently. You think people will think less of you, but, actually, they will think more of you if you live in your truth. It will transform you, open an opportunity to learn, and attract the people and help you need.

For instance, in a hospital setting, if there is something you do not know, say how to dress a wound, pretending you do will hurt the patient, as well as you. You will be fumbling around making a fool of yourself and battling inside. If you admit you did not get this properly in medical school, someone could offer to help and teach you.

- Imagine the presence of someone you respect, whose opinion you value

When you are in a moral dilemma, it is easy to fall into unethical behavior when you think no one would know. So, when you find yourself in such a position, imagine someone, say your child or your father—anyone whose opinion matters a lot to you—were there. Think, "How would my baby feel if they watched me do this?" "What would my dad think about the conversation I am having?" "Would my mum smile at what I am about to do?"

- Ask the help of a friend

You can ask another person to hold you accountable. It could also be a mutual arrangement of two friends seeking to walk in integrity. You can have them follow you up and be answerable to them about every action and decision. For instance, if you are struggling with doing what you said you would do, you can have them follow up if you actually did what promised yourself to. For instance, you said you would drive down to the countryside to unwind after a crazy week. They call or come over to make sure you are not watching movies on that day and watch you drive away.

- Be completely open to someone

Have a person whom you can tell everything. It could be a colleague at work, your best friend, or your spouse back at home. When we do not keep secrets to ourselves and at least have someone who knows us inside and out, it weighs heavily on whom we are and the choices we make. You do not want to go tell them that you left a patient calling out to you, to have a coffee break, so you will avoid doing that to the poor patient.

P.S.: Be careful who you choose to be an open book to. Not everyone can be trusted with that honor.

- Focus on saying less and delivering more

Be careful not to run your mouth. You see, talking too much may get you in trouble. You may get carried away and say things you do not mean, things which may portray you in a bad light. You may also make promises you cannot keep.

This is not to mean that you can't have fun or make conversation. Just be mindful of what comes out of your mouth. If you want to do something, it is better to deliver a surprise rather than talk about an intention you cannot fulfill.

- Commit to selflessness, the golden rule

Selfishness is the biggest barrier of integrity. So, choose to be selfless; live for others. Do unto others what you would love to be done to you. I bet you would not want anyone lying to you or treating you like crap. Practicing selflessness will give a boost to your personal integrity.

- Lead yourself

Be your own leader. This does not mean that you should not submit to authority. No, we are not talking about that. Leading yourself means you do what you need to do, what you know should be done without being swayed by the opinions of others. Trust me, if you were to follow people's opinions about what's right or what you should do, you will be running around like a headless chicken trying to please everyone and never really achieving it.

Do you remember the story of a man, his wife, and a donkey and all the opinions of the people they met? If you know this story, you remember that they ended up carrying a donkey; imagine doing that simply because someone thought it was unfair for them to ride on it.

So, drive yourself. Yes, ask for advice and guidance but be the one who makes the final decision on what to do. And remember: as you make your decisions, base them on your morals and values, not on pleasing people.

Integrity will make you a great person, and a great (successful, happy, and professional) nurse.

Conclusion

We have come to the end of the book. Thank you for reading and congratulations for reading until the end.

The 5 principles we have discussed in this book are tried, tested and proven to work. I live by them and I owe my 20+ years of a successful career in nursing to them. They will make you attractive in your profession; everyone—including yourself—will want and be happy in your presence. To the warm hearts who apply these principles, may you enjoy the success in your career that these principles will provide you.

I hope you use the many lessons in this guide. My YouTube channel is also chockfull of additional content related to nursing. Below is a link to my channel. Please subscribe, like, and share the videos that resonate with you.

https://www.youtube.com/channel/UCsv5zuZE_k15TzQ3y7f_G8Q/videos

If you found the book valuable, can you recommend it to others?

One way to do that is to post a review on Amazon.

Click here to leave a review for this book on Amazon!

Thank you and good luck!

Other Books By The Author

1. Everything I Never Told You: A Mother's Confession

https://www.amazon.com/dp/0998187496/

2. Positive Self-Parenting Solutions for Teenagers: Learning to Love Themselves from Scared Parents: Healing the post-traumatic stress in your life and Recovering you

https://www.amazon.com/dp/1974161617/

3. The Real Guide to Teenage Depression: Handling Teen Depression a book about what matters most for teen boys and teen girls

https://www.amazon.com/dp/0998187402/

4. Broken Teen Scars

https://www.amazon.com/dp/0998187410

5. operational Ugly truth

Made in the USA
Monee, IL
02 May 2024

57875678R00094